Re ow of *The GL Diet* Coo.

EASY SLIM-BY-SUMMER DIET

*'Welcome to the gourmet eating plan that
nourishes your senses as well as your body
while helping you lose a steady 2lb a week.'*
Zest, June 2006

Reviews of *The 7-Day GL Diet* (published Dec 2005)

THE NEW DIET SWEEPING HOLLYWOOD

*'It's the latest weight-loss plan sweeping the US with
Courteney Cox Arquette and Naomi Campbell reportedly
fans. J. Lo, too, is said to be a firm follower.'*
Reveal, 29 April 2006

*'The [7-Day] GL diet, combined with exercise,
is one of the best around.'*
Radio 1 *Newsbeat,* review of three diets, 19 January 2006

THE CAN'T FAIL 7-DAY DIET

*'Yes, it's a brilliant, no-panic party-dress diet but it's so
much more besides. It'll teach you how to stick cravings
right where they belong – out of your life!'*
Zest, January 2006

'The Crash Diet that's Healthy and WORKS!'
Elle, January 2006

'The GI has long been popular with celebs such as Kim Cattrall and Jodie Kidd – now they can follow a new improved version – the GL Diet … If you're determined to start 2006 with an improved diet, they don't get more user friendly than this one.'
Now, 29 December 2005

'Only The 7-Day GL Diet *proved to be an affordable option – incorporating healthy foods that aren't overly expensive.'*
Celebrity Diet Now, Winter 2005 (article comparing the cost of buying the food you need to follow the most popular diets)

Book of the Week – 'A fast and friendly plan for those always on the move, especially at this time of year.'
Grazia, 12 December 2005

'The GL diet is a more sophisticated version of the GI diet.'
The Times (3-page feature), 3 December 2005

'At last a book that takes low-glycaemic eating to the next level. Its beauty is in the simplicity and logic of its ideas. I will be recommending this to all my patients.'
Dr Andrew J. Wright, MBChB DRCOG MRCGP DIHom of The Complete Fatigue Clinic, Bolton, UK

Reviews of *The GL Diet* (published January 2005)

'The Glycaemic Load (GL) is the final part of the jigsaw. Testing for the GI (glycaemic index) of foods is a fantastic breakthrough, but it only gives half the true picture.'
Essentials (South Africa), September 2005

'Try the easy new GL Diet – everyone's talking about it!'
Essentials, June 2005

'Choice is back on the menu ... the GI diet has been superseded by a more sophisticated version: the glycaemic load (GL) ...'
The Times, 14 May 2005

'The GI diet is so last year. Take slimming one stage further with GL, a more sophisticated way of measuring the impact of food on your body's energy levels. Now you can love your lunch but still lose those love handles.'
The Times, 7 May 2005

'[The GL Diet] *is refreshingly clear and easy to understand; there's no high-tech scientific waffle ... it's a simple programme that uses a food selection system based on science, on fact not fad, but most importantly it's been designed to be practical and easy to follow.'*
Sunday Mail (Cyprus), 3 April 2005

'A good guide is Nigel Denby's The GL Diet ...
more useful ... more of a way of eating than a diet book.'
handbag.com, April 2005

*'An easy weight loss plan for life ...
simpler than GI and makes better sense ...'*
Evening Standard, 4 January 2005

*'The GL diet has been instrumental in helping me get back
to my pre-pregnancy weight. It's more than a diet though
and has just become a way of life. I've got so much energy
and don't have any of those food cravings I'd always
associated with diets and healthy eating – I love it!'*
Mishal Husain, News Anchor, BBC World News and News 24

THE GL DIET

MADE EASY

How to eat, cheat and still lose weight

Nigel Denby
Tina Michelucci and Deborah Pyner

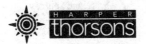

HarperThorsons
An Imprint of HarperCollins*Publishers*
77–85 Fulham Palace Road
Hammersmith, London W6 8JB

The website address is:
www.thorsonselement.com

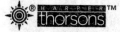

and *HarperThorsons* are trademarks
of HarperCollins*Publishers* Limited

Published by HarperThorsons 2006

3

© Nigel Denby, Tina Michelucci and Deborah Pyner 2006

Nigel Denby, Tina Michelucci and Deborah Pyner assert the
moral right to be identified as the authors of this work

A catalogue record for this book is
available from the British Library

ISBN-13 978-0-00-723336-6
ISBN-10 0-00-723336-1

Printed in Great Britain by
Clays Ltd, St Ives plc

This book is proudly printed on paper which contains wood
from well managed forests, certified in accordance with
the rules of the Forest Stewardship Council.
For more information about FSC,
please visit www.fsc-uk.org

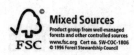

Mixed Sources
Product group from well-managed
forests and other controlled sources
www.fsc.org Cert no. SW-COC-1806
© 1996 Forest Stewardship Council

Contents

Acknowledgements

Thanks to Susanna, Laura, Chris and Sarah at HarperCollins for all their support and continued desire to help us spread the word!

A huge thank you also to our ever increasing band of diet freedom online club members gathered from our previous books (*The GL Diet Cookbook*, *The 7-Day GL Diet* and *The GL Diet*), our website (www.dietfreedom.co.uk) and by word of mouth. You continue to motivate us to motivate you, and to do the best we can to help you achieve your goals. Your honesty and feedback is invaluable and we find you all inspirational!

And last but not least our wonderful partners, families and friends who have been unstinting in their support of our mad working hours and passion for getting things right!

Thank you all so much.

Lots of love
Tina, Deborah and Nigel xxx

Chapter One
THIS DIET IS EASY

We've been there a thousand times – battling away at a diet we hate, feeling starving and fed up with eating crazy food combinations only to get to the end of the week and find that all that effort and misery has been in vain when we look at the dreaded scales and see a very disappointing result! Sound familiar?

Thank goodness we've found you! At last we can share with you what we and thousands of GL devotees have discovered – everything you could ever want from a diet and more!

Why is GL Different?

It's easy peasy

No counting, measuring or weighing! No getting up at
dawn to start scrubbing, peeling, dicing and juicing
weird fruit and veg concoctions (thank goodness!).

You can drop a dress/clothes size in a week or a month

It's entirely up to you how you use the diet, so you
can lose weight as quickly or as slowly as you want.
This is not a race but a permanent lifestyle change.
How healthy you are on the inside is just as important
as what you look like on the outside.

It's so flexible you can be as saintly or as devilish as you like

Of course, the more devilish you are the longer it will
take to shift the weight, but fear not – you will lose it.
You'll never have to avoid social occasions like the
plague because you can't eat anything but cabbage or
strange beans. The GL Diet allows for socializing
because it's based on real life, real food and real
people!

You can 'cheat' without guilt

In fact, we *positively recommend* a cheat or treat every
now and then. We all live in the real world with
temptation at every turn so we simply face up to it

before we indulge, make sure we enjoy it and then not use it as an excuse to give up. This is THE most important thing!

The GL diet is achievable and enjoyable ...
We'll never ask you to do anything we haven't done ourselves! In short, we understand what you are going through and how you got here in the first place.

... satisfying and safe
We hate feeling hungry. Starving ourselves and feeling miserable is a recipe for disaster: it's bad for you mentally and physically and never works in the long run.

GL is based on science (there are loads of research references later in the book if you'd like to know more), not hype.

The GL Diet is something you can follow forever. It's not just another 'quick fix' that will fail and keep you on the yo-yo diet treadmill. If you just want to drop a dress/clothes size for a holiday or special event then that's fine, but you can also take things more steadily if you have a lot of weight to lose or are looking to really change your eating habits to improve your health.

Why Do So Many Diets Fail?

Are we destined to fail because we are meant to stay a certain size? Of course not!

We've all tried diets that we hate, only to give up because it's just too hard, we don't like the food, we're constantly obsessing about food and we're STARVING! Ever gone to bed early because you've already eaten your allocated points/calories for the day? That's no way to live is it! But if it's familiar then remember …

**It's the diet that failed you –
you are NOT the failure!**

Some diets are such hard work there's no way you can stick to them, so you shouldn't feel guilty at all. We've all been there and got the T-shirt. If you've tried the myriad diets out there that are too rigid/ complicated/boring and full of false promises with no scientific basis whatsoever, toss them in the bin now!

GL isn't a quick-fix, faddy diet. It's a simple, healthy-eating lifestyle based on sound scientific research for people who want to lose weight and be healthy.

Sound too good to be true? Read on and see why we and so many other experts and dieters now trust and believe in low GL.

> *'Rather than being just a fad diet, GL represents a sustainable lifestyle choice, which is healthy and satisfying in the long term. The science is well founded, and has been talked about in academic circles for years, but now, as we are becoming expert nutritionists, we should all be more aware and conscious of GL as part of a healthy balanced lifestyle.'*
>
> **Dr David Haslam,**
> Clinical Director of the National Obesity Forum

How to Use this Book

There are lots of extra bits and pieces in the book to help you along your journey to find your own 'diet freedom' but **if you can't wait to get started you can go straight to the Plan in Chapter 4 or the 10-day Starter Plan in Chapter 5.**

For those of you who want the lowdown on the science behind the GL, Chapter 2 explains how your body uses the food you eat and how GL works with your body to help you stay in control of your food intake.

Chapter 3 looks at why the GL Diet is good for you – it's great at helping you to manage your weight but there are some incredible health benefits too.

Chapter 4 is the 'how to' planning chapter. You can jump straight to it if you want to skip the whys and wherefores. This chapter gives you everything you need to begin your journey to better health and 'feeling fabulous naked' – the low-GL way.

Chapter 5 has a 10-day Starter Plan for guidance to kick-start that weight loss. You can drop a dress/clothes size if you stick to the basic principles – you'll be amazed that it's not restrictive at all!

Chapter 6 tells you all you need to know to become a GL-savvy shopper. Our 'Angels and Demons' section gives you an idea of some of the best and worst foods GL-wise so that after just a few days you can cruise the supermarket aisles with confidence, knowing you are making the right choices.

Chapter 7 is all about keeping it real. We hope that, like us, you can't manage to be perfect all of the time! Cheats, treats or just plain slip-ups, we're all human and they will happen from time to time – it's human nature. Whether you choose to cheat, fancy a treat or make a mistake, this chapter will help with some damage limitation tips and guidance towards 'guilt free' indulgence.

If you're struggling for motivation, head for Chapter 8. We wrote this chapter to help you understand yourself and the best way to tackle making changes that fit in with you and your lifestyle.

It is proven that being more active helps you to lose weight more quickly. Not only that, but it also makes you feel fantastic. Chapter 9 is there to help you get moving, be more active and feel great. Don't panic – the emphasis is on being active and having fun, and it's not necessary to become a total gym bunny (unless you want to, of course!).

Last but not least, in Chapter 10 Tina and Deborah have been busy in the development kitchen creating more stunningly tasty, yet simple low-GL recipes. And wait for it … **ALL** of them take no more than **10 minutes** to make! It really couldn't be any easier to eat well.

We sincerely hope this book will free you from the dieting trap and make it extremely easy for you to get to your right weight and stay there. Together we have over 90 years of dieting experience – yes, we tried almost every diet under the sun until we finally worked out what actually works! Since then, between the three of us, we've been treating patients with weight and hormonal issues, working in dietetics, carrying out health and diet research, running diet trials in health clubs, developing recipes and eating plans for easy weight loss, running restaurants and writing books to help people like you. We really do know what works and what doesn't!

Everything you need to know is in this book. All you need to do is to get reading ... Enjoy!

Chapter Two

GL IN A NUTSHELL

This chapter examines the science behind GL. We look at how our bodies use food to make energy, and how that energy is used. We then go on to see how switching to low-GL foods works with your body to help you lose weight and keep it off. If you just want to get started on the diet, go straight to the plans in Chapters 4 and 5 – you can always come back to this section later.

A Bit about Fuelling the Body

There are three main nutrients in foods that give us energy in the form of calories – **carbohydrate**, **protein** and **fat** (alcohol also gives us energy but we'll put that to one side for a moment!). When we eat a meal, carbohydrates are digested and absorbed first, followed by proteins and then fats.

Carbohydrates are broken down into simple sugars (glucose); proteins are broken down into amino acids; and fats are broken down into fatty acids before being absorbed into the bloodstream.

The carbohydrates in foods affect our blood glucose and insulin levels the most. Insulin is needed by most cells in the body to act like a key and 'let in' the glucose from the blood so it can be used as fuel by the cell or so it can be stored. The amount of glucose that is floating around in our blood has to be carefully controlled within tight limits – too low and we will feel faint and dizzy; too high and our internal organs can be severely damaged. So it is the job of insulin to ensure that it keeps blood glucose levels under tight control.

Glucose is mainly stored in our muscle and liver cells to be used for energy as needed. Much of this stored energy is used when we are physically active. When the muscles and liver are full and can't store any more glucose, the only thing insulin can do is transfer the excess to other body tissues. **This excess of energy is stored as FAT**. Yes, those awful wobbly bits!

The carbohydrates in high-GL foods are very rapidly broken down to glucose and absorbed. This causes a huge rush of glucose into our bloodstream (glucose spike). The more glucose there is in the blood, the more insulin is produced (insulin spike). As a safety mechanism, insulin has to rapidly move this large amount of glucose flooding the bloodstream into our muscle and liver cells to be stored for later use. This can happen very quickly and cause blood glucose levels to drop suddenly (blood glucose crash). Don't worry if this seems complicated – you don't have to understand it all for the diet to work and we have a diagram on page 12 to show you what we mean.

When our blood glucose and insulin levels fall below a certain level, this triggers hunger signals in the brain. It tells us that we need to eat more because our blood glucose levels are falling quickly – as a result we crave more high-GL foods to satisfy the apparent hunger! What the brain doesn't realize is that we ate a doughnut (or any high-GL food) only an hour ago! This turns into a vicious cycle as the rapid fall in blood glucose prompts us to crave more high-GL foods – which actually caused the problem in the first place!

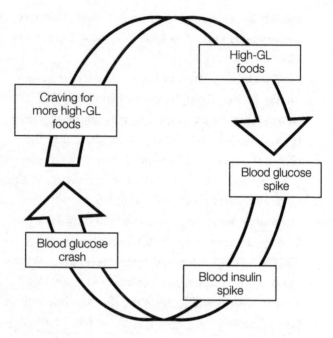

High-GL foods eaten = blood glucose spike = blood insulin spike = blood glucose crash = craving for more high-GL foods = weight gain!

Fear not – this vicious cycle can easily be broken.

The carbohydrates in low-GL foods are broken down to glucose and absorbed more slowly, causing only a small rise in blood glucose levels and a corresponding small rise in blood insulin levels. As a result, glucose is moved into our muscle and liver cells at a slower pace and blood glucose levels are more stable. Eating low-GL foods every three to four hours helps keep our blood glucose levels steady – meaning no glucose and insulin spikes, no blood glucose crash and (you guessed it) NO CRAVINGS AND OVEREATING!

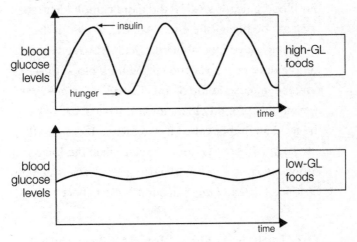

If we eat low-GL foods, we store less excess energy and blood glucose levels are kept stable, giving a slow-release, prolonged energy supply. This enables us to go about our activities with fewer cravings, feeling more balanced and of course ultimately **storing less fat**.

What Does High or Low GL Mean?

All foods that contain carbohydrate have an effect on our blood glucose levels – the more carbohydrate they contain, the bigger the effect. We can work out the effect they have in a laboratory setting by feeding people different foods and testing their blood to see how the glucose in the blood changes over time (we explain this properly in a minute). We can then give the food a number called its Glycaemic Index or GI (*see page 15*). Low-GI foods have a small but long-lasting effect on our blood glucose level whereas high-GI foods have a bigger but short-lasting effect.

The Technical Bit – How We Work Out the GI of a Food

GI is a scientifically proven method of categorizing foods according to how quickly the carbohydrates they contain are broken down and absorbed as glucose into the bloodstream. The Glycaemic Index or GI was created by comparing blood glucose levels of volunteers after eating different carbohydrate foods. Volunteers eat an amount of food that provides 50g of carbohydrate. Blood samples are taken from the volunteers at regular intervals over the next two hours to find out their blood glucose and insulin response to the test food. Each food is then given a number depending on how fast the body digested and absorbed the carbohydrate – the higher the number the faster the absorption. The number is called the food's Glycaemic Index (GI).

55 and under is low GI
55–70 is moderate GI

So far, so good.

Every food tested has a GI number telling us how quickly it is absorbed when we eat an amount that contains 50g of carbohydrate. But this is where the major problem with GI crops up. Different foods contain very different amounts of carbohydrate.

For example, to reach the laboratory test level of 50g of carbohydrate you would need to eat about 75g of pasta, so a small portion, BUT you would need to eat a whopping 500g of parsnips to reach the 50g carb level, and how often would we do that outside the laboratory? We love parsnips but not that much! We would generally eat about 100g of parsnips at any one time. So the GI number isn't based on realistic amounts of food that people usually eat in one sitting. The GI number you get for some foods like parsnips, watermelon and carrots, for example, is high, and if you just looked at the GI, these fine, nutritious foods would be deemed bad foods to be avoided! It's clear that there are problems with basing a healthy-eating plan on the GI of foods.

The Problems with GI

- The way the GI of a food is worked out doesn't always relate to the amount of food we actually eat at one sitting (remember the parsnips!).
- GI can be very confusing.
- If you base your diet on low-GI, some very healthy foods are excluded, such as carrots, watermelon, parsnips, pumpkin and broad beans to name a few. These foods contain little carbohydrate per portion and have a low GL.

GI gives us the first part of the story. It tells us that not all carbohydrates are equal; some are absorbed more quickly than others. But it doesn't take into account how much carbohydrate a food contains. This is where the Glycaemic Load or GL comes in.

The GL Makes Sense of the GI

The GL goes a practical stage further. It takes the GI rating we've just outlined, but then very cleverly (thanks to Professor Walter Willett of Harvard Medical School who came up with the equation) takes into account the amount of carbohydrate in a portion of food we would normally eat. So now we know the effect a normal portion of food would have on our blood glucose levels, and that's what gives us the GL rating:

- Foods with a high GI but with only a small amount of carbohydrate will generally have a low GL.
- Foods with a low or medium GI and a large amount of carbohydrate may have a high GL.

It's so simple and, more importantly, relevant to what we actually eat!

Foods rated using the GL do still get a number:

10 and under is low GL
11–19 is moderate GL

If you did want to count your daily Glycaemic Load (GL) for the first few days in order to gain confidence that you are on the right track, you would be aiming to have a GL score of 80 or under on a low-GL day. A high-GL day would be 120 or over. If you are overweight and inactive it's likely that your daily GL score is high and you are storing your excess energy as fat.

BUT don't worry – although we do give some basic portion guidelines and GL references, you don't have to count at all! Counting points, rigidly measuring and weighing foods is what turns us all off when it comes to diets. It's the bit that makes diets boring, boring, boring – and besides, who has the time? Counting can also reinforce the obsessive behaviour around food that got quite a few of us here in the first place! Pay attention to what you're eating and what your body is telling you. Once you've found your low-GL feet, it will all become second nature.

So What's Right about GL?

The Glycaemic Load (GL) gives you the whole story:

- The GL allows you to understand with confidence how foods will affect your blood glucose levels.
- The GL is based on carbohydrates in the portion sizes we usually eat, rather than the amount needed in a laboratory setting to work out the GI.
- The GL means far more food choices.
- The GL makes practical sense of the GI science. It's the final chapter in carbohydrate management and offers a real solution to weight loss.

There's one other thing that can affect the GL of a food. Let's get a reality check here. We don't often eat single foods at a time. When we eat a meal there's going to be a mixture of different kinds of foods, each with a different GL – so what happens then? Eating a food with a fairly high GL, such as white rice, could cause the spike in blood sugars we mentioned earlier. To avoid this you have two options. You can simply swap it for one of the recommended alternative lower-GL foods, like pearl barley. Alternatively you can just cut down the amount of it you eat and combine it with lower-GL foods, such as lentils or beans. This will give you a lower overall GL score for that meal. You can do this with all kinds of foods, which is one of the main reasons why the GL Diet is so flexible and fits in with the real world.

So now you understand:

- how our bodies deal with the food we eat.
- that high-GL foods perpetuate a vicious cycle of hunger and cravings.
- that the GL of a food is a more realistic measure of its effect on the body.
- that low-GL foods = more slowly absorbed = less hunger and less fat storage = weight loss.

Brilliantly simple, hurrah!!

All you need to do is read through the rest of the book and start enjoying healthy, low-GL foods, losing weight – and best of all, be able to keep it off forever as the GL Diet quickly becomes a way of life.

As serial dieters, we are all searching for our own elusive 'diet freedom' or 'freedom from diets'. The GL finally brings this within everyone's grasp without deprivation or hunger.

'I started with the GI, but found it contradictory and really confusing, then a friend told me about GL and I bought the book. I liked the fact that it's based on the GI but it makes more sense to me by taking the amount of carbs you eat into account.'
Christine from Bournemouth

'I was already GI-ing before GL-ing but it made a difference to me in that I lost the last half a stone I needed to.'
Caz from Rainham

'When I followed a low-GI diet, I really overate on pasta, which I now know has a high GL. Plus I was afraid of watermelon, which I love. Now I know watermelon is okay and it was ridiculous to avoid it. Those are just two minor examples of why I think GL is better! There are many more. I find the more I read the more I can apply my new knowledge to the way I eat. I'm so grateful for finding this new way of eating!'
Sheryl from California, USA
diet freedom online club member

The GL Diet is:

Science made simple – no magic wands or pseudo-science here!

A healthy eating plan you will want to (and can) follow forever.

Safe and suitable for all the family.

Bursting with loads of delicious food choices and recipes.

About having three meals and two snacks every day.

About making educated food swaps to change the types of carbohydrate you are eating – not about cutting out food groups altogether.

About eating for health – it is so much more than just another weight loss diet! You will feel fantastic on it – we promise you that.

A great way to live and eat healthily, so even if you stop following it you will come back to it – everyone does! The improvements in how you feel will make sure of that.

A common sense, no nonsense approach that will fit in with the way we live today in our fast-paced society.

Brilliant for foodies and 'fast' foodies alike!

So effective because it works *with* your body, not against it.

But most of all …

GL is about results – it's the perfect plan for losing weight because the weight comes off at the right rate for your body and so is more likely to stay off. There is *no* severely restricted start-up phase. The GL adjustments you are about to make are for good, and with the odd cheat and treat it is doable *and* enjoyable *and* will make you feel better than you have in years!

Chapter Three

THIS DIET IS SERIOUSLY GOOD FOR YOUR HEALTH

The GL Diet is not just a great eating plan for weight loss, it also embraces the importance of a healthy balanced diet and being physically active.

In this chapter we take you through some of the science and research that demonstrates how a low-GL diet:

- is beneficial to your health and wellbeing;
- improves the overall health of people with specific conditions;
- helps to improve symptoms of some common conditions.

Low GL and Diabetes

Because the GL Diet helps control blood glucose levels, it is beneficial to people with diabetes.

Type 2 diabetes is a condition where the body has lost the ability to tightly control the level of glucose in the blood. You'll remember that in Chapter 2 we talked about how it's the job of insulin to control blood glucose levels. People with type 2 diabetes don't produce enough insulin and/or it stops working effectively.

Choosing a low-GL diet for people with type 2 diabetes makes sense – glucose is released more slowly into the bloodstream and less insulin is needed in order to keep blood glucose levels steady. For people who aren't producing enough insulin, this means it's easier to keep blood glucose levels balanced.

The scientists certainly seem to agree with us. A team from Colorado State University in the US looked at the increasing prevalence of type 2 diabetes in urban areas of industrialized countries. The scientists found that over the past 200 years, the consumption of refined cereals and sugars has increased at almost the same rate as type 2 diabetes. The team concluded that the increased sugar in people's diets was clearly linked to higher insulin levels and the subsequent increase in type 2 diabetes.

Another study of over 40,000 health professionals reported that a high-GL diet increased the risk of developing type 2 diabetes. Similar findings were also reported by the American Medical Association who found that the women who ate more high-GL foods had a greater incidence of type 2 diabetes.

Both the European Association for the Study of Diabetes and Diabetes UK, the leading UK charity for people with diabetes, recommend a low-glycaemic, high-fibre diet as a means of maintaining good control of blood glucose levels and for helping to maintain a healthy weight.

A low-GL diet, along with regular activity, can help to control your diabetes and reduce your risk of serious long-term diabetes-related complications.

Even small changes to your diet can make a difference. Two large scientific reviews showed that a low-glycaemic diet has a positive effect on blood glucose control in people who already have diabetes, and that swapping just one high-glycaemic food for a low-glycaemic alternative can have a beneficial effect.

You can get more helpful information about diabetes from the UK charity www.diabetes.org.uk.

'The increasing prevalence of diabetes has huge social and financial implications for developed countries. With increasing incidence of conditions such as the metabolic syndrome, predisposing people to diabetes, the trend is even more worrying. I am convinced that making diet and lifestyle changes to reduce the risk or improve the treatment of diabetes is one of the most critical steps an individual can take. The GL Diet combines the fundamental principles of a healthy balanced diet with practical advice to help improve glycaemic control and long-term health.'

Sir Michael Hirst
Trustee and former Chairman of Diabetes UK

'I've had type 2 diabetes for 12 years. When I stick to a low-GL diet my blood sugars (and therefore mood, energy levels and so on) are easy to control. It's made life very simple, and even though I'm on the road a lot, I find that with only a bit of thinking ahead I have no problem sticking to it. I've also lost quite a bit of weight, which has pleased my diabetes nurse very much!'

Gary from Bedfordshire

Low GL and High Blood Pressure (Hypertension)

Hypertension is known as the silent killer – the condition can go undetected for years. Although high blood pressure can cause headaches, dizziness and problems with vision, the vast majority of people with high blood pressure have no symptoms at all.

Blood pressure is the force exerted by blood on the walls of your arteries when your heart beats. High blood pressure is a risk factor for heart attacks, strokes and kidney damage so it shouldn't be underestimated. Have your blood pressure checked by your GP or practice nurse every couple of years.

People who are overweight and have high blood pressure can expect to see a significant improvement in their blood pressure when they lose as little as 10 per cent of their body weight.

If you suffer from high blood pressure one of the most important things you can do is limit the amount of salt you eat. Studies show that many people with high blood pressure are 'salt sensitive', and they can better control their blood pressure when they eat less salt. Eating low GL means you naturally eat less processed food, which is where most of the salt in our diet is found.

Low GL and Heart Disease

Coronary heart disease occurs when arteries supplying blood to your heart muscle become narrowed by a build-up of fatty material. This slows down the supply of blood, and hence oxygen, to your heart. A heart attack occurs when the blood supply to part of the heart muscle stops altogether, usually because of a blood clot in the narrow part of the artery.

Eating a diet high in hydrogenated/trans fats and saturated fat, low in fibre and low in fruits and vegetables can contribute to the build-up of fatty material in the artery walls.

You can reduce your risk of developing heart disease by following the GL Diet. It has been found to be more effective than a low-calorie, low-fat diet. Evidence from around the world suggests that a low-GL diet may reduce the risk of heart disease in a number of ways.

In 1999 the World Health Organization and the Food and Agricultural Organization recommended that people in industrialized countries base their diets on low-glycaemic foods in order to prevent coronary heart disease, diabetes and obesity.

Several studies show that certain blood fats linked to heart disease are lower in people following a low-glycaemic diet. A low-GL diet is naturally high in fruits and vegetables, which are rich in antioxidants and have a protective role in heart disease.

> *'Is it worth getting nutrition right – and is it easy? We at HEART UK say yes – and yes! Simply eating well really is a good investment towards staying well.'*
>
> **Michael Livingstone**
> Director, HEART UK charity

Low GL and Female Health

Many women find that a low-GL diet helps to improve hormonally driven symptoms associated with premenstrual syndrome (PMS), polycystic ovary syndrome (PCOS) and the menopause.

From our experience, women usually feel improvements very quickly after lowering the GL of their diet and eating healthily. So stick to the GL Diet and monitor the reduction of your hormonal symptoms.

Polycystic Ovary Syndrome (PCOS)

This affects 10–15 per cent of women in the UK, although many don't even realize they have the condition. Symptoms include:

- Pelvic or abdominal pain from cysts on the ovaries
- Infertility, difficulty in becoming pregnant
- Recurrent miscarriages
- High blood pressure
- Acne
- Being overweight, rapid weight gain, difficulty in losing weight
- Baldness or excessive body hair
- Irregular periods

New research suggests that PCOS may be linked to raised levels of insulin in the blood, which stimulates the ovaries to produce too much testosterone. We discussed in Chapter 2 how eating high-GL foods causes high levels of insulin. Your body can become resistant to the effects of insulin and need more and more to be produced in order to have the same effect.

Carrying excess weight makes the symptoms of PCOS worse. A weight loss of 10 per cent is effective in improving symptoms.

Many dieticians working with patients suffering from PCOS recommend a low-GL diet to help control the levels of insulin produced by the body and to help with weight loss.

For more information and advice on PCOS visit the charity website www.verity-pcos.org.uk

'I've lost 6lb in two weeks so I'm thrilled. I have PCOS and endometriosis. The PCOS makes losing weight super hard and so the 6lb are even more exciting!

Emma from London
diet freedom online club member

'Thank you for the amazing things your diet has given me, like my life back! My close friend was diagnosed with PCOS, and when she described it to me I discovered that I had the same symptoms. So I researched diets and, lo and behold, I found the GL Diet. WOW! I've now been on it for two weeks and am a new person – I wouldn't go back if you paid me! I have energy and am no longer dizzy. The strangest change, though, is that my legs aren't as hairy – so exciting!'

Roma from Scotland

'I'd been gaining weight steadily since my diagnosis of PCOS. It felt like everything was going wrong at once and I was in a real downward spiral. I knew my diet wasn't great before, but it wasn't until I tried the GL Diet that I realized that what I ate could make such a difference. After just a week I had more energy than ever, and friends couldn't believe how well

I looked. I'm finally back in control of my
weight, and for the first time in two years I feel I
can influence how my PCOS affects me.'
Simone from London

The Menopause

The menopause is a time when a woman's fertility
declines. For most women, this occurs in their 50s,
although some women may face the menopause much
earlier or later than this.

As you go through the menopause your ovaries
produce less of the hormone oestrogen. This
reduction triggers the brain to release other hormones
in an attempt to make the ovaries work harder and
keep producing eggs. Symptoms such as hot flushes,
sweats, muscle and bone pain and poor concentration
are all linked to these hormone surges.

The GL diet can be beneficial to menopausal
women in a number of ways:

- Menopausal symptoms are hormone-related; the GL
  Diet better regulates the level of the hormone insulin in
  the blood.
- Stable blood sugars improve poor concentration and
  irritability.
- Many menopausal women find they gradually gain weight
  – the GL Diet is effective at helping to control weight.

- The menopause is a time when a woman's risk of heart disease increases; the GL Diet has been shown to be effective in helping to prevent heart disease.
- A low-GL diet can reduce the risk of breast and endometrial cancer in post-menopausal women.

'I first saw Nigel in his menopause clinic. I thought I understood GI back then although I clearly didn't really know what I was doing as I was getting nowhere fast. As well as trying to lose weight I wanted to control my mood swings and hot flushes and get a bit of my old spark back. Nigel taught me how to use GL, which made so much more sense to me than GI. He also talked me through the other aspects of my diet and lifestyle that would help me. In a few months I lost over two stone and my mood, energy and general feeling of wellbeing improved dramatically. I have now retired and see Nigel once a year to keep an eye on things, but after three years the weight is still off and I feel better than ever – there really is a life after menopause!'

Sheila from London

Low GL and Cancer

As with type 2 diabetes and some female health problems, some cancers are linked to our hormones. Breast, endometrial and prostate cancers have all been linked to the levels of insulin in our blood. Cancers of the digestive tract (stomach and colorectal) also seem to be linked to levels of insulin and other related compounds in the body. High levels of insulin occur when high-GL foods are eaten (*see Chapter 2*).

Research has also shown that a high-GL diet is positively related to the risk of colorectal, prostate, stomach, endometrial and breast cancers. This is most likely due to the effect high-GL foods have on our insulin levels.

Low GL and Child Health

The GL Diet has been shown to reduce food intake and body weight in children. Having a low-GL breakfast reduces the amount of food eaten for lunch, in both normal and overweight children. This could contribute to a significant reduction in overall energy intake and help combat the rising levels of obesity among children.

A low-GL diet has also been shown to be more effective than a low-fat diet in reducing BMI (body mass index) and body fat in obese adolescents.

> *'Yesterday I collected my two girls from school to find my eldest in a terrible state. She was white as a sheet, slightly clammy and shaking. It turned out that they'd had the biggest "dorm feast" ever, with the most sweets and fizzy drinks on record, a classic case of sugar overload. Needless to say, she wasn't very nice to be around – but two low-GL meals later, she'd come back down to earth and actually managed to sleep through the night. Thank you, Nigel, Tina and Deborah, for giving me the knowledge to cope with this kind of blood-sugar overload – it's making a huge difference to our lives.'*
>
> **Olivia from Scotland**
> diet freedom online club member

Low GL and Obesity

Being overweight isn't just about carrying around excess flab. The fatty tissue produces hormones that can make you susceptible to a number of chronic conditions – and the more overweight you are the greater the risk. Being overweight or obese increases the likelihood of you suffering from cancer, coronary heart disease, type 2 diabetes, hypertension, osteoarthritis and stroke.

The good news is that if you are overweight or obese, losing just 10 per cent of your body weight can reduce the risk of these chronic conditions significantly. The research showing beneficial weight loss on a low-GL diet is plentiful. Both adults and children show marked weight benefits and loss of excess body fat when following a low-GL diet.

Being on a low-GL diet doesn't reduce your metabolic rate as much as being on a low-fat diet – so at rest you are burning more calories on the GL Diet. This can only help with weight loss. GL dieters also report feeling less hungry than low-fat, low-calorie dieters, and actually eat less! Again, great for losing those wobbly bits.

'I've lost 7 stone since using the diet freedom website and books. It's a really logical way to lose weight and becomes second nature very quickly. It also makes you feel really good. The best thing, though, is that I've not regained any of the weight I've lost – this is a first as I'd yo-yo dieted my way through life up until this point. My confidence is much increased and it would be no exaggeration to say it has changed my life completely.'
Joe from Worthing

'In the two weeks I've been following this way of life, I haven't stopped eating and I haven't felt hungry. I've continued with a glass of red wine in the evenings, I've had the odd bit of chocolate and I've still lost 7lb. Can't be bad – I only wish I'd come across it sooner. Thanks to all involved with the books, the forum and all its members.'

Caroline
diet freedom online club member

'I thought I'd cheer myself up this morning by weighing myself, even though I hadn't planned to do so, and I'm absolutely delighted with the result! In the six-and-a-bit weeks since I started the diet I've lost a total of … 15lb! That's 6lb lost since my last weigh-in only two-and-a-half weeks ago. I'm taking as little exercise as ever, so I have to attribute my improved girth to the diet. This is definitely a very workable plan and fits in well with family life. It's easy to build meals around this sort of food, supplementing a basic low-GL core with higher-GL accompaniments and extras (such as potatoes) for the rest of the family. I'm very pleasantly surprised to find that it also helps me to lose weight!'

Astrid from Essex

Low GL and Concentration

Ever get the mid-morning or mid-afternoon sleepy feeling – when you just can't keep your eyes open? This can be a real problem if you're at work or school and supposed to be concentrating and firing on all cylinders.

Your brain relies on glucose as its sole source of energy – your muscles can use other things like fat and protein but the brain needs glucose. If your brain doesn't get enough then everything else slows down and that's why you feel sleepy.

Studies in the UK show that children who eat breakfast in the morning perform better and have better concentration in lessons. Choosing a low-GL breakfast like porridge or an oat-based cereal and eating low-GL snacks and meals throughout the day have a similar effect in contributing to this improved performance and concentration.

By following the GL Diet you give your body a steady supply of energy throughout the day, your brain has plenty of glucose to keep it going, and your muscles have plenty of fuel to keep you active too. The GL Diet is great for both body and mind!

Chapter Four

THE PLAN – HOW TO EAT

Time and time again we've seen diets burst on to the scene that promise miraculous weight loss but seem to overlook the body's basic need for a balanced diet – to achieve not only a healthy weight but also a healthy mind. We believe passionately that any lifestyle plan for weight loss should be a lifelong commitment to eating a healthy, balanced diet and being more active. However, we also understand that in the real world some people just want to drop a dress/clothes size before they go on holiday or for a special event. Either way, for any diet to get the thumbs up from us, the route to weight loss has to be sustainable, safe and enjoyable.

The GL Diet isn't just about switching to low-GL foods; it's also about making healthier choices whenever possible within the framework of a balanced diet. This is where we get down to the nitty-gritty. By following these guidelines you can be sure you'll get all the good nutrition you need to stay healthy and to lose any excess weight.

The GL Diet Guidelines

These are the things we think are important to focus on for a balanced diet and lifestyle, and we know they will work for you:

- Eat three meals per day plus two snacks.
- Don't go longer than four hours without eating.
- Eat no more than you can fit into your cupped hands at each meal.
- Swap high-GL carbs (like white bread) for low-GL carbs (like soy and linseed bread).
- Aim for two to three protein-rich foods each day – variety is the key.
- Base your snacks on low-GL fruit and vegetables.
- Try to eat five portions of fruit and vegetables every day.
- A moderate intake of fat is fine. Aim to eat mainly the healthier mono- and polyunsaturated fats such as olive oil and olive oil-based spread, vegetable and nut oils. Read

labels and avoid harmful hydrogenated/trans fats hidden in many food products. Some foods are now labelled as containing 'non-hydrogenated fats', which is great.

- Be aware of salt hidden in many processed foods and don't add it to recipes or at the table.
- Drink six to eight glasses of fluid each day – water is best.
- Try to be more active and make it fun – aim for 30 minutes each day.

Most of us know the basics of healthy eating. However, choosing the right foods can be daunting, so we often put our heads in the sand and carry on regardless. But you can relax – our recipes and food lists take care of all that so you can get on with your life, look and feel great and still enjoy fabulous food.

Sometimes understanding a few of the facts behind the healthy eating guidelines we suggest can make it a bit easier to see why we should all be making some changes, so this chapter explains why the guidelines are important. If you feel confident that you understand good nutrition and just want to get started, skip this section and go to Chapter 5 for the 10-day starter plan.

Three Meals and Two Snacks

Eat something when you wake and then every four hours. This helps to get you into a regular routine with eating. You won't go hungry, and meeting your nutritional needs is much easier.

Eat Low-GL Carbs at Each Meal

Low-GL carbs include vegetables, fruit or whole grains. These help you to feel fuller for longer, so you're less likely to get hunger pangs and reach for the biscuit tin. They are also good sources of insoluble fibre to keep your bowels healthy, and regular and soluble fibre which help lower cholesterol and promote healthy gut bacteria.

People who regularly eat whole grains have a reduced risk of heart disease, type 2 diabetes and some cancers. Whole-grain carbohydrates like oats and pearl barley have a low GL (*see GL food lists in Chapter 11*).

It's the Carbohydrate-rich Foods that Make the Difference

If a food contains little or no carbohydrate then it will have a zero GL and no effect on your blood glucose levels. If your portion size of carbohydrate-rich foods is bigger than the one we recommend in the GL food lists, the GL will be higher.

Swap High-GL Foods for Low-GL Foods

This is where you can make a big difference. Low-GL foods will even out your blood glucose levels, helping you feel fuller for longer and reduce cravings for carb-rich, sugary and starchy foods. Fewer hunger pangs mean you're much less likely to overeat and put on weight.

You'll get the greatest benefit from swapping foods that contain the most carbohydrate and have the highest GL like white breads, sugary breakfast cereals, overcooked white pastas, sugar-laden cakes, pastries, biscuits and sweets, white rice and large white potatoes.

Make it a Way of Life – Keep It Simple Sweetie (KISS)

Making your diet and food complicated just adds to the stress of the whole thing, and that is not what the GL Diet is about at all. Following the plan should be a breeze. All the recipes in Chapter 10 take 10 minutes or less – and they are *so* easy to make! You don't need a Michelin star to have a go and you certainly won't be slaving over a hot stove for hours! They are just simple 'back to basics' recipes that taste great.

Think Natural

We're passionate about cutting back on highly processed foods as many are full of sugar, salt, additives and unhealthy hydrogenated/trans fats.

If you cook with natural ingredients from scratch you know exactly what goes into your body; you're in complete control with no hidden 'nasties' to worry about. By making your own meals you can increase the variety of foods you eat and have more 'cheats and treats' using alternative, low-GL ingredients.

We wanted to recommend some healthy, natural, low-GL treats for you to buy but sadly we couldn't find any that came up to our exacting standards – so we made our own! Look out for the diet freedom range of natural 'guilt-free' treats, from brownies to flapjacks, cheesecakes to carrot cake and ice cream, coming soon to a store near you! See www.dietfreedom.co.uk, our online health and diet club, for our latest product launches.

Eat until You're Satisfied, not Stuffed

Eat slowly and listen to your body. Stop eating at the first hint of feeling satisfied. Don't feel guilty about leaving food. Following our portion guides closely will help you not to put too much on your plate in the first place. Aim to finish all your vegetables/salad and leave the carb-rich food until last.

- Only eat as much as you can fit in your cupped hands at each meal.
- Try to be consistent about the amount of food you eat at each meal time and never skip meals.
- Use the Angels and Demons guide to the goodies and baddies *(see Chapter 6)*.
- Don't be a slave to the kitchen scales – you might want to weigh a recommended portion size once to see what it looks like but that's it. **There's absolutely no need to weigh everything you eat!**

Enjoy Your Food

Plan your week and you won't get caught out. Look at your work and social diary for the week ahead, and try to plan for potential meals out, long working days, social events and so on. Go shopping with a list and stick to it, and have a selection of meals to choose from for the entire week so you don't get tempted to forget the plan when you haven't got the right foods in.

Chapter Five

THE 10-DAY STARTER PLAN

We've put together a 10-day guide to help you create the perfect plan for *you*. The GL Diet is flexible and fits in with real life, unlike other 'eat this on day one or else' diets, which just don't work. Use the 10-day guide to fit around *your* life and know you are doing the right things and making positive changes.

Having no flexibility in a plan can be a real barrier to ever getting started, and we can't have that! Remember that you can be very flexible, have a really easy time and still lose weight and start to feel the benefits of the food swaps you are making.

We suggest that, if possible, you start the plan over a quiet-ish weekend. On Friday, stop off on the way home and pick up something tasty for breakfast, some fresh juice and fresh fruit. Then when you get up on

Saturday morning, enjoy your lovely low-GL breakfast, make your plan for the next ten days (remember to factor in any social occasions) and then clear your cupboards of the high-GL 'baddies'. You can then go shopping for your low-GL 'goodies'. Do this while you're not hungry, and feeling strong and full of resolve for the journey ahead!

Of course if your quietest day is a Tuesday, start then! Don't let this become another excuse not to start. We have one member who started with a dinner party for eight and has never looked back!

Remember, this isn't a 'diet' – it's 'diet freedom', your passport to freedom from dieting forever! *Enjoy* and tell yourself and anyone else that you are *not* on a diet but have started to make informed judgments about what you eat instead.

If you're hungry, eat. Keep small snacks handy – better an apple at 11am than a blowout at 1pm! Focus on the health benefits of low GL as the primary target and the weight loss will follow naturally without you thinking about it too much. We really want you to feel that you're not dieting or doing anything restrictive, as restriction equals tension, and tension equals rebellion and we all know what follows that, don't we? So, sit and relax, take a deep breath in, hold for a count of four and breathe out slowly. Repeat three times and then say out loud, 'I am not on a diet – I am making positive choices for my health and enjoying my life to the full.' It's really helpful to repeat this whenever you can – looking in the mirror at the same time reinforces the message to your subconscious mind. Another great time to do it is just before you fall asleep as this is when your brain is most receptive to positive affirmations. In other words, your brain will take it on board and believe it, keeping you on track! Any sceptics out there should try it – it works a treat!

Remember, if you stick to the plan you should drop a clothes size in the next 10 days. Now you're ready to get started. Happy food swaps – enjoy!

Notes on the 10-day Plan

Where the following are mentioned, the recommended portion sizes are:

WOMEN: oatcakes/crispbreads – up to two, bread – one slice (so an average day may be either two oatcakes/crispbreads *or* a slice of bread but not both)

MEN: oatcakes/crispbreads – up to four, bread – up to two slices (so an average day may be either four oatcakes/crispbreads *or* two slices of bread but not both)

- In our experience, some people find it difficult to metabolize grains and to lose weight while eating them. If this applies to you, try cutting them out until you reach your target weight. You'll need to make sure you get plenty of fibre from vegetables, beans and pulses – psyllium husk is a great alternative fibre provider available from health food stores.

- Natural low-GL sweeteners are a new and evolving area and are not widely available at the time of going to press. The best on offer at the time of writing is agave syrup, although it is expensive. We recommend that before you get started you visit www.dietfreedom.co.uk and look under the heading Low-GL natural sweeteners, where you will find an up-to-date list of our recommended products with stockists for all your low-GL sweetening needs. As there are a few of our recommended foods that are quite new and not widely available yet you will also find a list of these with stockists on the website.
- You can find all our recommended low-GL foods and portion guidelines in our food lists in Chapter 11.

Day 1

Breakfast

How about a leisurely cooked brekkie of two or three slices of lean grilled bacon (or bacon substitute for veggies) and two poached eggs? Low GL and satisfying. Try out the Naughty Weekend Breakfast recipe on page 152.

Mid-morning Snack

Two squares of dark chocolate with 70 per cent or more cocoa solids make a great snack You can get some great varieties now such as orange, peppermint or ginger.

Lunch

A couple of rye crispbreads, such as Ryvita, or sugar-free oatcakes with a low-GL topping such as a vegetable or fish pâté make a good lunch option.

Mid-afternoon Snack

A handful of dried apple makes a great portable snack. You can also buy apple crisps from some stores – they are surprisingly nice as a treat now and then!

Helps towards your five a day!

Dinner

Fancy a rice dish tonight? Try pearl barley as a lower-GL alternative or mix some lentils with the lower-GL brown or wild rice.

Day 2

Breakfast

For a special late Sunday brekkie we like a little
smoked salmon either in an omelette or on some
toasted rye bread with cream cheese. Mmmmmm!
Counts as a portion of heart-friendly oily fish.

Mid-morning Snack

A small handful of dried pears? They are more readily
available nowadays – check out the health food stores
if you can't find them in the supermarket.
Helps towards your five a day!

Lunch

A beefsteak tomato, halved, with flesh scooped out
and mixed with cream cheese or houmous and any
leftover salad.
Helps towards your five a day!

Mid-afternoon Snack

A rye crispbread such as Ryvita is ideal – easy to eat
and versatile. Try with a thin spreading of sugar-free
peanut butter (most peanut butters have added sugar
so check the label).

Dinner

Sunday lunch/dinner is no problem. A few swaps is all
it takes – use sweet or new potatoes instead of white;
roast a rainbow of vegetables or sweet potatoes
brushed with olive oil. Use organic vegetable bouillon
for gravy as it won't have nasty hydrogenated/trans
fats in it.

Day 3

Breakfast

Fill a tall glass with half fruit juice (with bits = more fibre and lower GL) and half water. Combining fruit and veg juices, diluted with water as above, will make sure you pack a good nutritional punch. Experiment! Toast a slice of rye bread and spread with a smear of olive oil-based spread or butter and enjoy.

Helps towards your five a day!

Mid-morning Snack

Too busy to remember to have your snacks? Set the alarm on your mobile to remind you! A couple of sugar-free oatcakes with cream cheese are a good filling choice.

Lunch

Vegetable soup is great for lunch. You could make your own (*see recipes in Chapter 10*) and take to work in a Thermos or buy fresh cartons from the supermarket (about half a standard carton is a portion).

Helps towards your five a day!

Mid-afternoon Snack

Cut yourself a matchbox-sized piece of cheese.

Counts as one of your three daily portions of dairy for healthy bones.

Dinner

A 120g portion of oily fish, such as a fresh tuna steak, counts as one of your two recommended portions for the week. See our recipe for zingy Tomato Tuna (page 203).

Day 4

Breakfast

Not very hungry? Have a refreshing sugar-free smoothie – either buy in or make up your own (*see Chapter 10 for ideas – we highly recommend the Cinnamon Banana Smoothie!*).

Helps towards your five a day!

Mid-morning Snack

Some crudités and a houmous dip? You can buy carrot batons with dips in some coffee bar chains now and most supermarkets too. The washed bags of sweet baby carrots are fabulous to keep in the fridge at all times to munch on.

Helps towards your five a day!

Lunch

If you are making pasta, remember that cooking it 'al dente' helps keep the GL lower. Stick to a handful of pasta and fill up on veggies or salad instead.

Mid-afternoon Snack

A 30g portion of unsalted nuts has been shown to reduce hunger later in the day – try almonds as they're great for lowering cholesterol!

Dinner

Soya protein and Quorn are low GL so if you are vegetarian there are lots of choices. You can substitute either for any of the meat in the recipes whether you are a veggie or not!

Day 5

Breakfast

Late for work? Keep plenty of sugar-free bran flakes in
your cupboards, add a swirl of agave syrup, some
chilled milk and *voilà!* The perfect low-GL brekkie in
a shake!

Mid-morning Snack

You can't beat a large crunchy apple!
  Helps towards your five a day!

Lunch

Reduced-sugar beans on a slice of low-GL toast make
a good lunch option. Choose a bread such as Burgen
soya & linseed, pumpernickel or rye.

Mid-afternoon Snack

Any fruit you fancy – an orange or pear perhaps?
Whatever is in season will taste the best.

Helps towards your five a day!

Dinner

When you're choosing meats, select the leanest cuts
and ask for any visible fat to be trimmed. Try the
Seared Strips of Beef with 'Cabbaghetti' recipe (*see
page 182*).

Day 6

Breakfast

You can't beat old-fashioned porridge oats when there's a nip in the air! It only takes a nanosecond and you can cook it in the microwave if you're in a rush. In warmer weather try our Fruity Cool Porridge recipe (*see page 145*) or give our lovely Creamy Coconut Porridge a whirl (*see page 146*).

Mid-morning Snack

A small handful of dried apricots makes a great portable snack if you fancy something sweet.
   Helps towards your five a day!

Lunch

Sandwich on the run the only option? Look for the darkest, grainiest bread available and leave the top piece, making it an 'open sandwich'.

Mid-afternoon Snack

Maybe a couple of satsumas? Nice and easy to eat.

Dinner

Chicken and turkey are good lean meat choices – go organic if you can. See our choice of chicken and turkey recipes in Chapter 10. Turkey Sweet 'n' Spicy Stir-fry *(see page 198)* is one of our favourites!

Day 7

Breakfast

We love a tablespoon of natural, sugar-free yoghurt
with chopped fresh or dried fruit first thing – it makes
you feel alive! Remember, the more natural the better.
Try our Easy Granola Yog Pot recipe on page 150.

*Counts as one of your three daily portions of dairy
for healthy bones.*

Mid-morning Snack

A small handful of mixed seeds makes a great snack –
you can buy them in tubs to keep handy or take to
work.

Lunch

If you go for tinned soup, check the label and make
sure it doesn't contain hydrogenated/trans fats or
added sugar. Avoid potato- and pasta-based soups.

Mid-afternoon Snack

Cottage cheese is a good dairy source and tastes great with chopped fresh peach, pineapple or mango.

Counts as one of your three daily portions of dairy for healthy bones.

Dinner

When choosing fruit and veg, think colourful and try to 'eat a rainbow' every day. Try our great Mediterranean Couscous recipe on page 180.

Day 8

Breakfast

Overslept and have no choice but to grab and run this morning? Take a nutritious, natural, low-GL muffin with you (*see recipes on pages 148 and 171*).

Mid-morning Snack

A small handful of sugar-free dried cranberries fits the bill as a portable snack – do check the label though, as they often have loads of sugar added!

Helps towards your five a day!

Lunch

If you need to grab and run, a shop-bought sugar-free smoothie and a filled pitta or wrap are your best bets (look for the darker pittas and wraps rather than the highly processed white ones which will have a higher GL).

Mid-afternoon Snack

Individual cheese portions make great snacks – check out the myriad of choices in your supermarket.

Counts as one of your three daily portions of dairy for healthy bones.

Dinner

Prawns are so versatile. You can keep them in the freezer and defrost quickly for a fast and friendly lunch or dinner. They are also great in stir-fries. We love the Leafy Prawn Salad recipe on page 156.

Day 9

Breakfast

Grapefruit makes a brilliant brekkie. The latest
research says it is *so* good for your health, especially
the red ones! We like to halve them, smear over some
agave syrup for sweetness and leave in the fridge
overnight to infuse.

Helps towards your five a day!

Mid-morning Snack

A small handful of any unsalted nuts is a nutritious
and filling snack *but* they are all loaded with calories
so don't overdo it!

Lunch

Two poached eggs on toasted rye bread will help fill
you up and keep those cravings at bay.

Mid-afternoon Snack

Guacamole (made from avocado) makes another great oatcake or rye crispbread topping. You can either buy it ready-made or blend your own.

Helps towards your five a day!

Dinner

No time to cook tonight? All the recipes in this book take only 10 minutes or less! They are completely painless to throw together – honest! So get to the recipe section now!

Day 10

Breakfast

Any leftover fruit need using up? To make a colourful fruity breakfast salad, wash or peel, chop and toss in a bowl, top with a tablespoon of crème fraîche or natural, sugar-free yoghurt and sprinkle with a few chopped nuts.

Helps towards your five a day!

Mid-morning Snack

A banana – choose the firm, green, stripy ones as the ripe ones have a much higher GL.

Lunch

Wash some iceberg lettuce leaves, keeping them intact, and lay flat. Layer on some lean meat or cheese, add a teaspoon of mayo or dressing, roll up into a wrap and eat – quick, easy, tasty and low GL!

Mid-afternoon Snack

A kiwi fruit (not over-ripe).

Dinner

We all adore Indian food! You can still have
international cuisine, fear not. Avoid the rice and naan
and enjoy with a large salad and veggies instead.

Diary of a diet freedomer!

'Started lowering my GL today … woke feeling ready to start eating well … I've made my plans for the week, bought a few things so am well stocked up! Threw out any high-GL foods in the cupboards that I know are not good choices and felt very virtuous afterwards! Breakfast was porridge with a dollop of crème fraîche and some fresh, chopped strawberries swirled in – felt very NON diet, liked it a lot. Large glass of ice cold water and a cup of tea later, feeling great and still surprisingly full! Clipped pedometer thingy on and walked to work for first time in years, so well on my way to my 10K steps challenge today! Bought bottle of water on way and finished it before I got to work.

'10.45: not hungry but ate a couple of dried apricots I had stashed in my office drawer and a handful of toasted seeds with a glass of water and a cappuccino.

'Out for lunch with the girls in the office – had a lovely ham and mushroom omelette with a big tomato and rocket salad (couldn't finish it actually, stopped when I'd had a "cupped handful" and realized I was full!) and a small fresh orange juice. Persuaded everyone to take the stairs instead of the lift back to the third floor! And it's normally me who's first to the lift! We all puffed a bit, but will get less each time.

'Afternoon tea break was easy. Had a cup of tea and three squares of the lovely individually wrapped 70 per cent dark choc I'd bought with me – heaven! Ate it slowly and savoured the taste which is growing on me, especially now I know about the nasty trans fats in my normal choc bars! Friend Emma said "What a great idea" about the choc – so I may be a trendsetter! No-one guessed I was on a diet – whoops, sorry – eating healthily! Normally by 2.30pm I'm falling asleep in my chair and can't concentrate as I've had lots of white bread and sugar-filled milk chocolate by this time, but amazed that I feel really alert and can get on with my work without feeling brain dead and just staring at my computer screen in a daze.

'Feeling *so* virtuous at 5.30. Literally ran down the stairs and had a brisk walk back home feeling very smug, picking up tuna and tomatoes for tonight's dinner. Checked pedometer – WOW! Only another 200 steps and will be at 10K! Am shocked at how easy it is.

'Threw together spicy tuna dish* and a salad in less than 10 minutes. I was full again before my plate was

* See recipe on page 203.

empty (this is unheard of for me). Drank a couple more glasses of ice cold water instead of my usual two glasses of red wine, with a splash of fresh lime in it, a sinless spritzer! All that extra water really made me feel more energized. By the time I went to bed I'd done 10,197 steps and felt great – this whole low-GL thing really could work – it isn't at all like being "on a diet" – in fact, no-one would even guess …'

Chapter Six

ANGELS AND DEMONS

Okay, so we're aiming to avoid the demons (bad foods) as far as we possibly can, especially if we have a lot of weight to lose. However, if you really, really fancy a demon, have it, enjoy it and don't feel bad about it – you'll see throughout the book that an occasional cheat is actually encouraged! But we also need to stress here that your diet should be made up of mainly angels (good foods). You may notice after a wee while that you become more angelic by nature and a halo appears as if by magic.

Below we give you the main demons and angels in each food group but you will also need to become familiar with the full A–Z list of low-GL foods with recommended portion sizes and corresponding GL values in Chapter 11.

Some foods are so low in carbohydrates per serving that they are impossible to test for their GL – most berries for example – but as they are low in carbohydrates they will have a low GL so are included. Foods that are made up of less than 5 per cent carbohydrate have a minimal impact on your blood sugar levels. These include some dairy products, fats and oils, meat and fish.

As GL testing is ongoing we aim to give you the most up-to-date information available, so any newly tested foods – both generic and branded – after publication of this book can be found on the members section of our website (www.dietfreedom.co.uk).

All of the following weights are cooked weights if the food is normally eaten cooked (unless otherwise stated).

If you make up your own recipes and food combinations using low-GL ingredients you can increase your food choices and variety tremendously. Food manufacturers and supermarkets are slowly beginning to catch on but you still need to be a bit of a detective when it comes to getting the best choices into your basket. That's exactly why we wrote this chapter, to make shopping low-GL style as easy as pie (low-GL pie of course!).

Breakfast Cereals

General Points

Here's a good opportunity to make a low-GL choice
and kick-start your metabolism when you wake. Many
commercial cereals have added vitamins and minerals.
However, they often contain a hefty dose of sugar and
are highly processed before they reach our breakfast
bowl, so avoid these. You can use any milk you like
from cow's and goat's to soya. A portion of cereal is
around 30g (dry weight) or 2–3 tablespoons.

Demons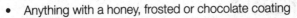

- Anything with a honey, frosted or chocolate coating
- Most flakes and crispie-type cereals, which have added
  sugar

Angels

- Porridge oats (use old-fashioned oats, not sachets of
  instant porridge)
- No-added-sugar bran flakes or bran sticks (you can
  liven up porridge and bran breakfasts with some
  chopped fresh or dried fruit and/or natural, sugar-free
  yoghurt)

Add a drizzle of low-GL agave syrup to the milk to
sweeten the above bran brekkies ... mmmm!

Shopping Tips

See www.dietfreedom.co.uk for stockists of all low-GL
breakfast cereals, natural sweetening alternatives and
recommended ingredients and products. You can also
buy raw ingredients from the health food store and
make up your own sugar-free muesli with oats and
chopped dried fruits such as apricots, pears, apples
and strawberries.

Breads

General Points

A portion size of 30g is approximately one slice from a
medium loaf. A good guideline to stick to would be
no more than one slice of bread per day for women
and two for men while trying to lose weight. Gluten-
free breads tend to have a higher GL as they are often
based on corn. Generally the darker and grainier the
bread, the lower the GL.

Demons

- Any white or highly processed bread

Angels

- Soya and linseed bread such as Burgen
- Pumpernickel or sourdough rye bread
- Stoneground wholemeal pitta bread ('stoneground' means it is less processed so the GL should be lower)
- Stoneground wholemeal wraps (rare to find but freeze well, so stock up!)

Other lower-GL breads include: spelt multigrain or whole grain (just because it is brown or 'wholemeal' doesn't mean it will be low GL as it can still be highly processed – look for stoneground wholemeal).

If a recipe calls for flour as a coating, experiment with oat flour, spelt flour, oatmeal or low-GL breadcrumbs, and if you need a thickener in place of white flour, try arrowroot or spelt flour.

Shopping Tips

Most of the above are now widely available in high-street supermarkets. If you're lucky enough to have a good local bakery they will often produce some fantastic low-GL breads made from rye or spelt. If you're really stuck, look for the darkest, grainiest bread you can find.

More Demons

- Crumpets
- Pikelets
- Scotch pancakes (you can make your own lower-GL versions of pancakes and blinis with buckwheat flour, *see page 188)*
- Croissants
- Pastries

Cakes, Biscuits and Sweets

Sadly, most commercial brands are chock-full of sugar and often contain hydrogenated/trans fats … bleugh!

Demons

- Sugar-filled cakes, scones, buns, doughnuts, fancy cakes and slices, cream cakes, biscuits and virtually all commercial sweets!
- Beware 'diabetic friendly' or 'low-carb' sweets and pastries – they often contain polyols such as maltitol or xylitol which can have a severe and unexpected laxative effect!

Angels

See our healthy recipes in Chapter 10. After two years' development we are very proud to say we have launched our own delicious range of diet freedom natural 'guilt-free' treats, including a cinnamon-spiced carrot cake, moist chocolate brownie and an oaty flapjack. These all have a low GL, with no added sugar (sweetened with natural fruit extracts), contain no hydrogenated fats, are wheat free, GM free, high in fibre and suitable for vegetarians (the brownie is also gluten free). Keep updated on stockists and further product launches at our website at www.dietfreedom.co.uk

Desserts and Puddings

Again, most commercial brands are full of sugar and hydrogenated/trans fats.

Demons

- Sugar-filled cheesecake, gateau, sponge puddings, crumbles, meringues, pies and pastries.

Angels

See our healthy recipes and alternatives in Chapter 10, or if you must have a pud and don't want to make your own, try our diet freedom brownie or carrot cake (see above) warmed with a spoonful of good quality ice cream – a divine angelic treat! The flapjack makes a great granola-type topping crumbled over yoghurt and chopped fresh fruit too. We also cut our diet freedom cakes into four pieces and eat them as snacks throughout the day.

Crackers and Crispbreads

There are good and bad versions of these.

Demons

- Highly processed white crackers
- Corn crispbreads
- Rice cakes
- Anything that looks pale and uninteresting!

Angels 😇

- Rye crispbreads (such as Ryvita)
- Sugar-free oat cakes

There are now loads of whole-grain crispbreads available with ever more imaginative ingredients such as dark rye, sesame, spelt, roasted onion, sunflower seeds and oats …

Rice

General Points

White rice is a high-GL food – if you choose to eat it, keep to a small portion – about 75g when cooked (50g dry weight), and have it as an accompaniment rather than the largest part of the meal. You can also mix it with beans and pulses to lower the GL of your meal without reducing the overall quantity, or use pearl barley as an alternative as it has a GL of only 8 for 150g! Many of our readers and diet freedom online club members are getting very creative now with pearl barley, making 'barleyotto' and any number of beany combos! In fact, they are so creative we are truly inspired.

Demons

- White, basmati, jasmine, short-grain, long-grain, risotto-type rice

Angels

- Pearl barley
- Wild rice
- Brown rice
- Couscous
- Bulgur wheat
- Butter beans, haricot beans, cannellini beans
- Pulses/lentils

Shopping Tips

All the above are available at good supermarkets and health food shops.

Pasta

General Points

Try and keep your pasta to smaller portions – about 100g when cooked (about 50g dry weight). Think of pasta as an accompaniment rather than the largest part of the meal.

Cook pasta 'al dente' (firm to the bite) – the longer it is boiled the higher the GL rises!

Gluten-free corn pasta has a moderate to high GL, depending on the brand. Mixing beans and pulses with pasta will enable you to have a bigger portion and lower the GL of the overall meal.

From our own experience and feedback we feel that the amount of pasta you can eat and still lose weight varies significantly from one person to the next – so start with smaller amounts and see how it affects you.

All weights refer to cooked weight unless otherwise stated. Pasta almost doubles in weight when cooked, so 50g of dry buckwheat pasta is almost 100g when cooked. Each type of pasta will vary a little, and fresh pasta usually absorbs less water during cooking than dried. If you have to have white pasta, look for the egg-based, fresh versions.

Demons

- Tinned or overcooked white pasta.

Angels

- Wholewheat pasta
- Mung bean noodles

- Buckwheat pasta and noodles (sometimes called soba noodles)
- Ravioli filled with meat, vegetables or cheese
- Chickpea pasta

Try 'Cabbaghetti' in place of pasta – shredded cabbage and other shredded lightly boiled or steamed veggies – delicious!

Shopping Tips

Most of the 'angels' listed above are available in supermarkets – try the chiller cabinet for fresh egg-based pasta, chickpea pasta and fresh filled pasta like ravioli and tortellini. For soba and mung bean noodles, try an oriental supermarket. We've hunted down some great pasta alternatives, so check out the '♥ shopping' page at www.dietfreedom.co.uk

Other Grains, Beans and Pulses

General Points

Pearl barley, bulgur wheat and couscous can be used in place of rice or pasta to lower your GL for the day.

Beans and pulses are a fantastic source of fibre, and most have a low GL, so experiment with beans and pulses in stews, soups, salads and pasta dishes. You don't have to buy dried beans and spend days soaking and boiling. Canned beans are just as good and supremely convenient. Drain and rinse well if they are canned in brine or buy versions without added salt or sugar whenever you can.

Demons

There are no 'major' demons here, although most whole grains should be eaten in moderation when in weight-loss mode and supplemented with lots of lovely veggies, salads and fruit. When they're 'whole' they have health-giving properties – it's when they're processed to death that the GL rises and you lose the health benefits.

Angels

- Pearl barley
- Couscous/bulgur wheat
- Butter beans, cannellini beans, haricot beans, pinto beans, chickpeas, mung beans, kidney beans, broad beans, blacked beans
- Baked beans (choose reduced-sugar/salt varieties)
- Lentils/split yellow peas
- Sprouted beans, pulses, grains
- Wild rice, brown rice

Other grains you could try: quinoa, whole rye, whole wheat and buckwheat kasha.

Shopping Tip

Most items are available at good supermarkets. You could try a health food shop for some of the more unusual grains, beans and pulses.

Vegetables and Fruits

All angels, not a real demon among them!

General Points

The vast majority of fruits have a low GL. In the food lists in Chapter 11 we've given the GL for a 120g portion – this amount should fill the palm of your hand. Not all fruits have a GL rating – this is because they're very low in carbohydrates. Berries are very low GL and a brilliant choice. Stick to firm fruit – if it's soft and over-ripe the GL will be higher, especially with bananas and tropical fruits.

A little note about potatoes: large potatoes have quite a high GL. Three or four baby new potatoes are fine. Try mashed or baked celeriac, sweet potato or yam instead – these have a much lower GL but still give you a mashed potato fix. Mashed cauliflower with a little butter, black pepper and mustard is something you must try as it makes a fantastic low-GL topping to pies, and you'll be surprised at how good it tastes – we promise! Recent research has shown that cooked, refrigerated potato with added vinaigrette (such as potato salad) has a much lower GL than just cooked, hot potato!

Try to eat a rainbow of coloured vegetables every day to get a good variety of antioxidants, vitamins and minerals. Make sure you get at least three portions of veg and two of fruit per day if you can. The portion sizes in the food lists in Chapter 11 apply to cooked vegetables (obviously you will sometimes eat raw veggies).

Shopping Tip

Most fruits and vegetables are available from supermarkets or greengrocers but you may have to look a bit further for more unusual varieties. For extra fresh fruit and veg visit 'pick your own' farms (another big tick in the 'activity' box!) and farm shops for seasonal produce with that lovely just-picked freshness!

Dairy Foods, Alternatives and Eggs

There are no real demons in this section either, as natural dairy foods, eggs and alternatives with no added nasties are pretty angelic! Just follow the guidelines below and you'll be sure you're not taking in too much saturated fat.

General Points

Dairy is an excellent source of protein and calcium – three dairy portions like a pot of yoghurt, a small piece of cheese and a third of a pint of milk will give you enough calcium for the day. Dairy foods can be high in fat and calories – choose lower-fat versions whenever possible.

Non-dairy milks and yoghurts can make an important protein and calcium contribution for people who don't eat animal products. Make sure they're enriched with calcium. Yoghurts vary a lot in content – stick with sugar-free natural versions. Or preferably add your own fresh fruit to natural yoghurt (such as bio or Greek).

Cheese is a great source of calcium but often quite high in fat. Choose lower-fat and reduced-fat hard cheeses, and stick to 75g per day as a guideline maximum. Lower-fat cheeses include cottage cheese, Edam, feta, goat's cheese, Gouda, mozzarella, ricotta and reduced-fat hard cheeses.

Choose your favourite milk – cow's, unsweetened soya, almond, oat, goat's or sheep's. Aim for a maximum of half a pint a day. Skimmed or semi-skimmed milk is a good choice while in weight-loss mode. Eggs are another 'superfood', and one a day is now regarded as fine for healthy individuals.

Crème fraîche, sour cream, natural good quality ice cream, cream and mayonnaise are all fine in moderation. See the low-GL food lists in Chapter 11 for full details.

Shopping Tips

There's a good selection of dairy products available at supermarkets. You may need a health food shop for a greater variety of non-dairy milks and yoghurts.

Fats and Oils

General Points

All fats and oils are low GL because they don't contain carbohydrates.

Demons

The top demon is hydrogenated or partially hydrogenated fat. Although butter has a bad reputation as it's a saturated fat, it's probably far less harmful than the many low-fat spread alternatives we've been encouraged to consume in its place for the last 20 years or so. Many of these spreads contained hydrogenated fats. The hydrogenation process produces trans fats, which health researchers are now linking to heart disease and cancer. As a result of this, governments throughout the world are now introducing either a complete ban or drastically limiting the amount of hydrogenated/trans fats products are allowed to contain.

The many olive oil-based spreads now available make a healthy alternative to butter. Olive oil is a healthy fat but still high in calories. Aim for no more than a dessertspoon of olive oil or olive oil-based spread a day. Look for spreads that say non-hydrogenated fats or virtually trans fat-free. It's also a good idea to keep your intake of saturated fats to a minimum and concentrate on the 'healthy fats' such as olive oil.

Angels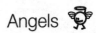

Our top angels are:

- Olive oil, a great healthy choice to use in salad dressings and as your usual cooking oil
- Olive oil-based spreads – great for baking and frying
- Nut oils – great for salad dressings
- Groundnut oil has a higher 'smoke point' than many other oils, making it great for stir-fries

If you're keen to know more about oils, we cover the subject extensively in *The GL Diet Cookbook*.

Shopping Tip

Oils and spreads are available from all supermarkets, health food shops and specialist online shops.

Meat

No meat is 'bad' per se. It's how it's used and processed that can be alarming! We've got no demons here, but a few guidelines.

General Points

All meat is a very good source of protein. Being very low in carbohydrate, the GL for all meat is zero. That's not to say you can turn into a meat fiend! Remember to trim any visible fat from meat and remove the skin from poultry.

As a rough guide, a portion of raw meat should be about the size of a deck of cards. For you number crunchers, this is about 75–120g of red meat or 100–150g of poultry. Try to stick to no more than three portions of red meat per week.

By choosing unprocessed, fresh meat you are treating your body to a good quality protein without additives or fillers. By choosing free-range or organic, you go that step further by considering the welfare of the animal too.

Angels

- Chicken – a versatile low-fat meat. Remove the skin.
- Beef – an excellent source of iron. Remove visible fat and try not to add any extra while cooking.
- Turkey – low fat, and can be used in the same way as chicken. Turkey mince is a good lower-fat alternative to red meats.

Other meats you can use: liver, pork, ham, gammon, bacon, game (pheasant, venison), duck and ostrich, kidney and good quality high-meat-content sausages (90 per cent plus).

Shopping Tip

Meats are available from supermarkets and butchers, but you may need to go to a specialist for game meats. Farm shops and farmers' markets have locally produced meat. Much of it is free range, outdoor reared or organic and you can really taste the difference.

Meat Alternatives 👼

If you're vegetarian or vegan it's important that you
include sufficient protein from a wide variety of
sources. Soya and Quorn are good low-GL choices.
Also include some beans, pulses, nuts (and dairy
foods or eggs if you eat them) to ensure you get a
wide variety of different types of protein. Try to have
two different vegetarian sources of protein every day.
An average portion would be about 100–150g.

Fish 👼

Like meat, fish doesn't contain any carbohydrate and
so the GL for all fish is zero. The omega-3 fats found
in oily fish are great for taking care of you and your
heart. They make the platelets in your blood less
sticky and help prevent arteries from clogging.
Approximate uncooked portion sizes are: white fish
150–200g; all oily fish/tuna and salmon/shellfish
120g–150g. Aim to eat three portions of fish per week,
with at least one being oily fish.

Our Favourites

- Salmon – fresh, smoked or canned: one of the best choices for omega-3 fats.
- White fish – cod, plaice, coley, hoki, monkfish, sole, tuna: all fabulous!
- Mackerel and herring – great sources of omega-3 fats. Can be eaten fresh, smoked or canned.
- Fresh tuna is also counted as an oily fish. Canned isn't because of the cooking process it goes through.
- Sardines, pilchards, kippers, crab, lobster, prawns, scallops, anchovies and caviar! – all goodies

Shopping Tips

If you're lucky enough to have a local fishmonger, he'll have a great choice of fresh fish and seafood. Supermarkets have the most commonly-eaten fish and seafood in the chiller cabinet – it's even better if they have a fresh fish counter. Frozen fish is a really great standby, and as fish is caught and frozen so quickly, it's actually one of the freshest options!

A Word about Organic and Local

It's not always possible to buy organic or local – it can be expensive, and not all of us live near a farm shop! However, organic is better whenever possible. Organic (or home-grown!) veg won't have been treated with pesticides. Free-range and organic eggs are available everywhere now, and we highly recommend you buy these over the battery caged hens' eggs for both your conscience and your health. We're all trying to help ourselves get healthier and fitter, and we can feel even more virtuous when we take animal welfare and the environment into consideration too.

Memory Box

- Follow a healthy balanced diet based on plenty of fruits and vegetables and lean protein.
- Think of carb-rich foods like bread, potatoes, pasta and rice as accompaniments to a meal rather than the main part.
- Choosing lower-GL versions of foods like bread, potatoes, pasta, rice and desserts will have the biggest effect on the success of your low-GL plan.

Chapter Seven
CHEATS AND TREATS

As well as being passionate about health and nutrition, we're also passionate about food – we love to eat! We still have the occasional slip-up, cheat or treat. Just like you, we live in the real world where nobody's perfect all of the time. Let's face it – the few people who are almost perfect are actually quite scary!

The point is that life keeps us all pretty busy and we have to take some short cuts. It's also human nature that if we're told we can't eat something, all we think about is how we're going to eat it without anyone knowing. That's what this chapter is all about – making room for cheats and treats so they're just part of your plan rather than being something you have to feel guilty about!

How Often is it Okay to Cheat?

We like the idea of the 80/20 rule. This means watching what you do 80 per cent of the time and relaxing a little 20 per cent of the time. Some people adopt this by being more careful during the week and then a bit less cautious at the weekend. The important word here is control. If you don't feel you're able to relax without going completely overboard then it's probably better to wait a little while before you try.

The 80/20 rule is something to consider when you've reached your weight-loss goal. If you're very focused on weight loss right now, then it's obvious that the more treats you have the longer it's going to take you to achieve your target.

Whenever you do have a treat there are some really useful tips you can use to make sure it's just that – a treat and not a guilt-ridden, hurried binge which leaves you feeling hopeless and a failure.

- **Focus on what you're eating:** make the food the main focus of your attention.
- **Put the food on a plate:** don't eat chocolate or a biscuit, for instance, from the packet. Take the portion you feel comfortable about eating, put it on a plate and move out of the kitchen to eat it.

- **Don't eat your treat in front of the television:** sit at a table so you're not distracted by the television.
- **Take your time:** really savour every mouthful of your treat. If you rush it you'll be far more tempted to go back for more.
- **Keep a record of treats:** Instead of pretending a treat 'didn't happen', take responsibility for it, acknowledge that you had and enjoyed it – even note it in your diary so you keep track of just how often you are indulging.

What Counts as a Treat?

A treat is giving yourself permission to enjoy a food you don't normally have all the time. It might be a couple of squares of milk chocolate or a glass of wine. A healthy relationship with treats is something that people who don't have a weight problem understand very well. You're aiming to be able to have a small amount of a treat and say to yourself, 'That was delicious, I really enjoyed it and because I didn't over do it hasn't ruined my eating plan.'

You might have a cheat when you're pushed for time or just don't have the inclination to cook from scratch or walk to work. Cheats are things that often trip us up when we're dieting. It's very easy to think because you haven't done X, Y and Z that the rest of the day has also been a disaster. If we have issues around food, we're very good at focusing on the negative and missing all the good things we've achieved.

If you know you're going to be stuck at work until late and won't want to cook when you get home then with a bit of thought you can cheat your way around that situation perfectly well. If you follow general low-GL principles and use the 'Angels and Demons' section in Chapter 6, you will soon see that you can buy low-GL ready-meals which won't pile on the pounds. Keep a stock of frozen vegetables and fruits in the freezer and you can have a balanced, healthy meal in minutes straight from the microwave.

Similarly, if you've been getting your daily 30 minutes' activity by walking to work and for whatever reason just can't manage it one day that's fine. Just make a conscious note that throughout the rest of the day you need to try and use the stairs more often, or pop out for a walk at lunchtime, even if it's just for 10 minutes. Cheats are all about making the best of a difficult situation – careful cheats = damage limitation.

Other Times You Want to Treat or Cheat

Going out for Dinner

Eating out is great. It's social, relaxing and a chance to let someone else do the cooking. See it as a treat and enjoy it! Use these tips to help you stay in the driving seat.

- Don't skip meals throughout the day to compensate – you'll be so hungry when you get there you may be tempted to make poor choices.
- Order some water while you read the menu – this will help take the edge off your appetite.
- If the bread basket arrives and you really fancy a piece, choose the grainiest, darkest option, but if there's only white bread or you know that one piece will lead to another and another, skip it and focus on what you're going to order instead.
- Ask for sauces and gravy on the side so you can have just a little.
- Order extra veggies or salad instead of potatoes.
- Decide whether you want to have a starter and main course or a main course and dessert – try not to have all three.

- Watch the wine. As well as giving you extra 'empty' calories your reserve will drop a little with each sip and you'll be more at risk of having a blowout!

Dinner at a Friend's House

When our nearest and dearest have taken the time to cook for us, the very last thing we want to do is make a scene about what they've prepared because it doesn't suit our diet. Try letting them know in advance that you're being careful about what you eat at the moment. They'll probably ask you if there's anything you are trying to avoid or eat more of – a good tip is just to ask them to prepare some extra veggies or salad so you can load up with these.

If you're faced with a high-GL extravaganza, remember it's only one meal and not a catastrophe. Imagine your plate is divided into four quarters. Use two of the quarters for vegetables or salad, a quarter for the protein part of the meal – the meat, fish or chicken if you eat it – and the last quarter for the carbohydrate. This way of balancing your plate, along with the 'no more than you could fit into your cupped hands' rule, will limit the damage even the highest-GL meal could cause.

Working Away

Staying in hotels can be a nightmare when it comes to food. Lots of temptation and all those dinners with clients and colleagues can prove difficult. Try to book a hotel with a swimming pool and take your cossie with you so you can get some extra activity in the evening – that way you won't have to spend quite as much time in the hotel bar! Pack some snacks with you for during the day. Dried apricots, seeds and unsalted nuts are available in handy packs and will make it easier to avoid biscuits and pastries at meetings. And use the eating out tips, above, when ordering meals.

Holidays

We all need a break from routine from time to time, and the most important part of any holiday is that you relax and have a good time. You can use the break from routine to stop a holiday turning into a weight gain. Whether it's a city break or a beach holiday, introduce plenty of walking into your day. Limit your indulgence to one meal a day. Choose a sensible breakfast and lunch and make dinner the time when you relax more, and use the eating out tips above to help you when you are eating in restaurants.

It's probably sensible to aim for weight maintenance while you're away – weight loss isn't always realistic when you're on holiday. Plan ahead for when you get back – have a menu in mind for the first couple of days and some low-GL foods in the freezer for the first night's dinner so you can get straight back on track.

Christmas, Easter and Special Occasions

Just like holidays, these events come round year after year, and there's no getting away from the fact that they tend to revolve around food and drink. If you accept that they're coming and plan accordingly, they really don't have to be a nutritional nightmare. Work out exactly how many people you're going to be entertaining, plan the menu and shop only for the amount of food you're going to need – piles of leftovers are likely to end up in one place and one place only! Here are a few tips:

- Experiment with lots of different vegetable side dishes – you can produce a table laden with lovely food without it all having to be rich and full of fat and sugar!
- Instead of the usual nibbles like sweets, chocolate and crisps, use dried apricots, pears, apples and strawberries, unsalted nuts, seeds, dips like houmous and crudités or toasted wholemeal pitta bread.

- Watch the booze – set a limit for how many drinks you will have and stick to it. Have at least one glass of water between each alcoholic drink or have a sugar-free soft drink instead.
- Follow the 'eat every four hours' rule to stop you getting over-hungry.

'Just had a dinner party and the whole menu was low-GL style. Nobody knew!'

Andie from Harlow

In Chapter 8, 'Getting Your Head Right', we talk a lot about realistic expectations and planning being crucial elements of any successful weight-loss or healthy-eating plan. You might think because we're now talking about cheating and treating that we're contradicting ourselves. In fact, expecting that from time to time you'll want a cheat or to cut the odd corner, and then planning for those times, is at the very heart of what we discuss in Chapter 8.

More than anything else we want you to adopt a low-GL diet for the long haul. If you're not prepared to enjoy another meal out or holiday or Christmas then that just isn't realistic and you're almost guaranteed to fall off the wagon and find yourself feeling guilty – which is the recipe for a relapse.

Remember:

- **A lapse** is a slip – it's normal and everyone has them.
- **A relapse** is a return to old ways and is what keeps so many people stuck in their own diet trap.
- **The art of a successful lapse is not letting it turn into a relapse.**

'This is a wonderful freedom from the bad four-letter "d—-" word, and I haven't weighed or counted anything (fats, sugars, calories, sins, points) for four months, and feel so much better about it all. My weight loss is slow, but then, we're not talking crash diets here. We're talking a way of life that's sustainable through all life's ups and downs, of which there are new ones every day! I need to lose about three stones, but more importantly, at the vast old age of 63, I need a way to avoid the increasing chance of diabetes and heart problems, arthritis, high blood pressure and so on. I'm so grateful that I found this way of eating.'

Karen from Glasgow
diet freedom online club member

'I think the way the eating plan makes you feel is as good as any weight loss it brings! When I stick to the GL Diet for a few days it definitely makes my cravings go away, and I've also found it helps with PMS symptoms.

Helen from Cheshire
diet freedom online club member

'It's great to not be on a dreaded diet, not have to fork out £5 a week for someone to tell you you've put 2 pound on that week. It's just a new way of eating. I now find very much to my amazement that I don't crave, don't want to stuff my face and when I actually taste those yummy looking cakes, choc etc I don't actually like the sweet cloying taste. GL is dead easy when you eat out, no forward planning like when I did slimming world. If you were on a green, carb day and went for a meal that wasn't rice or pasta based you were snookered. When I think of all the huge amounts of pasta and potatoes I consumed on that 'diet' I go yuk! It has improved my mood greatly as I'm not filling up on refined ready made rubbish.'

Ruth from Lancashire
diet freedom online club member

Chapter Eight

GETTING YOUR HEAD RIGHT

Congratulations! Chances are that if you've got this book in your hands you've already decided that the GL Diet is the way forward, and that this way of life is going to be a critical part of achieving and maintaining a healthy weight.

Now before you get going we really urge you to take just a little time to plan and prepare for change. Also, to stop and think about some of the things which might get in your way of changing or trip you up. In our own experience, and from what Nigel's patients and our army of diet freedom online club members tell us, a little preparation goes a long, long way towards success.

Changing long-held behaviours like eating and activity levels is not as easy as it first appears, but a

few simple strategies can really increase your chances
of making the changes you want.

- **Set your goals:** decide on what you want to change
  about your lifestyle.
- **Plan your action:** choose what actually needs to
  happen so you can achieve your goals.
- **Beat the barriers:** adopt actions to overcome the
  things that stop you changing your lifestyle.
- **Seek support:** find other people to help you stay on
  track.
- **Resist relapse:** get straight back on track when you
  start to waver, and don't feel guilty or wallow in despair
  thinking you've 'blown it' – you haven't. And always
  remember that the only failures in life are those who
  don't try …

The next section will help you put your action plan
into practice, and get you on the road to a new
healthy low-GL lifestyle.

Setting SMART Goals

SMART goals will help you decide on the changes you want to make and then to translate these into goals you work towards. SMART goals will significantly improve your chances of getting where you want to be and of staying there. Make your goals SMART:

Specific: clear and simple, not general. Instead of saying, 'I'll eat less junk food,' say, **'I'll take a packed lunch to work every day and cook from scratch at least three nights a week.'**

Measurable: you must be able to see that your goal is being achieved. Instead of saying, 'I'll get more active,' say, **'I'll achieve at least 10,000 steps a day on my pedometer.'**

Achievable: you must make sure your goal can actually be reached. Instead of saying, 'I'll eat chickpeas every day because they're low GL,' say, **'I'll experiment with one new recipe a week which includes different types of beans and pulses.'**

Realistic: don't set a goal you have no hope of achieving. Instead of saying, 'I'll never eat chocolate again,' say, **'I'll enjoy chocolate and will choose chocolate with at least 70 per cent cocoa solids which won't cause a peak in my blood sugars.'**

Time-specific: don't say, 'I'll get around to trying some new recipes one day,' say, **'I'll choose two new recipes to make this week, plan what I need to buy, go to the shop today and make sure I have everything I need.'**

Planning Your Action

Okay, your goals are set and they're SMART, but how are you going to achieve them? Let's say you want to aim for five portions of fruit and vegetables every day. There are lots of strategies you can use to achieve this goal.

Change the quantity
You could decide to add dried or fresh fruit to your porridge at breakfast to give an extra portion, or you could add some cherry tomatoes to your lunch box, or an extra portion of veg with dinner.

Change the frequency
If you eat fruit on only three or four days a week at the moment, you could decide to increase this to at least one piece of fruit as a snack every day.

Change the type

Instead of ordering a sugary dessert at the restaurant, you could decide to order a fresh fruit salad, and how about asking for extra veg to help fill you up?

Small changes really will add up to make a difference. The more changes you make, the more your confidence will grow and the more you'll love what happens to your body.

Beating the Barriers

If you've made your goals SMART and planned your actions carefully, you've every chance of success. But life has a funny way of putting things in our way, and some of those barriers can all too easily lead us down the road to a relapse. Anticipating the barriers will give you all the power you need to smash the barriers to a pulp.

Some of the most common barriers are:

No time to shop

We love online shopping. Most of the major supermarkets provide this service, which as well as saving time makes it much easier to resist some of those high-GL foods because they're not sitting on the

shelf, right under your nose, yelling 'buy me, buy me!'
We have some great guidance on mail order food
companies on our website www.dietfreedom.co.uk

No time to cook

Well, first of all, every recipe in Chapter 10 is designed
for simplicity. We've worked tirelessly to come up
with some fantastic, fast and friendly recipes, all taking
only 10 minutes or less! You can also use the days
when you do have a little more time to cook some
meals in advance and freeze them. Stock up on
freezer staples like sauces and soups and use healthy
convenience foods like canned pulses and frozen
fruits and vegetables.

Can't cook, won't cook

You don't have to be a trained chef to eat a healthy
low-GL diet. We love an easy life and that's why all
our recipes are quick and easy, with no fancy cooking
methods. We also write all our instructions in plain,
simple language. The art of great food is good
ingredients simply put together with a little
imagination.

Short of cash

Buying fruit, veg, meat and fish in season is always
cheaper. Keep an eye out for special offers and bulk
buys but only if you can store them and will use them.

Local markets, farmers' markets and food co-ops are great not only for quality and freshness but also for bargains. You could even think about an allotment which will give you all the fresh fruit and veg you need and be a great way to get some gardening activity in! Even the most un-green-fingered of us can grow herbs and lettuce in a window box or pot, and it's very easy to grow the likes of tomatoes and courgettes – they just need light, food and water, like most of us!

Food likes and dislikes

We all have foods we don't like, and just because a food you hate is on our food list YOU DON'T HAVE TO EAT IT! However, if you haven't tried some of the foods we recommend, that's different. Make a plan to include a couple of new foods each week and see how you go. The only rule we have on this is, you don't know that you don't like it till you try it!

Seeking Support

Trying to change your lifestyle will be much easier if you have a little support for the 'bad days'. Here are some suggestions.

- Join our diet freedom online club at www.dietfreedom.co.uk. We have a great community, with members from all over the world, and busy forums where there's always someone around to give you just the boost of confidence and enthusiasm you need. Tina, Deborah and Nigel are always calling in as well to answer questions and give encouragement. Members also receive a regular newsletter with new recipes, GL information, tips and health news. We're also building the biggest online low-GL recipe database available, with over 400 recipes at the time of going to press!

- GL is a great way of life for everyone. There's no reason why the whole family can't eat low GL. If they're not interested in losing weight that's fine too. Just give them slightly bigger portions – simple!

- If you've got a colleague at work who's interested in your low-GL lifestyle, see if they'd like to join you. You can take turns to prepare low-GL lunch boxes for each other and also go walking together at lunch time to build up your steps.

Resisting Relapse

Each of us, all of our diet freedom online club members and all of Nigel's patients have slipped up at one time or another – it's completely normal when you try and change any aspect of your life, and we promise you that you too will slip at some time. Whether it's one meal, a whole day, a week or the whole of the Christmas holidays, it's vital to accept that your diet won't be perfect *all* of the time.

From time to time we also have those days when it seems like it's all a bit too much. Stress at work, kids playing up and hormonal changes can leave us feeling vulnerable, and it only takes one of our old triggers to let everything slip. The odd slip here and there isn't going to wreck all your hard work – try to keep it in perspective. But be aware of your triggers and plan another reaction rather than eating.

Phone a friend

When you feel that a lapse is on the horizon a quick call to someone who knows you're trying to change could be all you need to refocus.

Log on to the forums

There's always someone in our chat room who'll have been there and bought the T-shirt. A trouble shared …

Do some walking

Removing yourself from the situation is a great tactic. It gives you a few minutes to take stock of the situation and decide on a constructive course of action.

Get some R & R

Relaxation techniques can be really useful for resisting a relapse. Yoga, massage or even a good long bath are great 'me time' activities – making time for yourself is vital.

Try a temptation tamer

Some of these are our favourites. Others have been contributed by our fantastic readers and members. Just pick a couple that ring a bell for you and keep them handy for moments of temptation.

Tried and Tested Temptation Tamers

Junk food = lousy mood

Kitchen pickers wear bigger knickers

Junk food junkie or health food hero?

Bad for me, bad for my bum/hips/tum/love handles

Just one will be the tip of the iceberg

Do what I always did and I'll get what I always got

Will eating this make me feel better or worse?

No thanks, I just don't eat that anymore

I want to be slim and feel great more than I want to eat that …

Success Measures

Now you've done all that preparation let's think about how you want to measure your success. After all, it's a dead cert that you're going to be successful!

Body Weight

It's probably fair to say that for most of us the scales are pretty important at telling us how well we're doing. We strongly recommend if you choose to weigh yourself that you pick another success measure as well and follow the rules below.

- Weigh yourself a maximum of once a week.
- Use the same scales every time.
- Weigh at the same time and on the same day every week.
- Work out your average weight loss over a month rather than focusing too much on what happens each week.

Pick one of the following success measures to accompany weight measures.

Waist Circumference

Abdominal fat, or the fat we carry around our middle, is a good indicator of our risk of heart disease. You can measure your waist circumference once a month. Place a tape measure around your waist, level with the upper edge of your hipbone – don't hold your breath! As you make progress it's useful to know that a loss of 1cm around your waist is equal to about 1 kg (2.2lb) of body fat loss.

Waist Circumference Classifications

Please note: South Asians living in the UK have a higher prevalence of diabetes than Caucasians so the recommendations for waist circumference are more stringent, as shown in the table.

	Healthy level	Level 1: increased health risk	Level 2: substantially increased health risk
Men	Less than 94cm (37 inches)	More than 94cm (37 inches)	More than 102cm (40 inches)
South Asian men	Less than 90cm (36 inches)	More than 90cm (36 inches)	
Women, including South Asian women	Less than 80cm (32 inches)	More than 80cm (32 inches)	More than 88cm (35 inches)

Clothes Size

We all know that our clothes can indicate when things are going well and not so well. Well, now it's official. Researchers at Glasgow University have recently been able to predict our health risk by the clothes size we buy. Some of the clothes sizes mentioned here refer to waist measurement – you need to be aware that clothes manufacturers measure waist circumference differently to the way we described previously. Increased health risk is equivalent to a trouser waist size of 34 inches for men in the UK and a UK dress size 14 for women. Substantial health risk is equivalent to a waist size above a 36 inch trouser for men and a UK dress size 16 for women.

Body Mass Index

Body mass index or BMI is a number that measures the relationship between your weight and your height and offers an estimate of your risk of weight-related disease. If you're a number-cruncher and would like to calculate your BMI manually, just follow these three steps:

1. Work out your height in metres and multiply the figure by itself.
2. Measure your weight in kilograms.

3. Divide the weight by the height squared (the answer to step 1.)

For example, you might be 1.6m (5 feet 3 inches) tall and weigh 65kg (10 stone). The calculation would then be:

1.6 x 1.6 = 2.56. BMI would be 65 divided by 2.56 = 25.39.

Or if you hate maths, check out the BMI calculator on www.dietfreedom.co.uk

Classification of Weight Categories Using BMI

BMI	Category
Less than 18.5	Underweight. You may need to gain weight.
18.5–24.9	Normal weight. Aim to stay the same.
25–29.9	Overweight. Weight loss may help your health. Avoid further weight gain.
30–39.9	Very overweight. Your health is at risk. Losing weight will improve your health.
More than 39.9	Morbidly obese. Weight loss is essential to improve your health.

Current research suggests that the healthiest BMI is 21 and that a BMI above 28 doubles your risk of illnesses and weight-related death. However, BMI is not a perfect measure and cannot distinguish between fat weight and muscle or lean weight, and it doesn't account for age or gender. So use BMI as a guide and not the 'Holy Grail'.

Weight-loss Targets

Whether you have a lot or a little weight to lose, the end target can seem a million miles away. When Nigel works with his patients he always encourages them to set weight-loss targets in 10 per cent milestones. This makes each target very achievable, and each milestone also brings with it a whole host of health benefits. Let's say you currently weigh 15 stone (95kg). A 10 per cent weight loss is 21lb or 1½ stone or 9.5kg. If you lose an average of 2lb (approximately 1kg) each week that will mean you reach your first target in just 11 weeks or around three months. After losing 10 per cent of your starting weight you will obviously feel great but will also have:

- reduced the likelihood of dying of a diabetes-related illness by 40 per cent;
- halved your chance of dying from an obesity-related cancer such as breast cancer or cancer of the colon;
- reduced your blood pressure;
- reduced your cholesterol levels by 10–15 per cent;

- improved your level of HDL (good) cholesterol;
- halved your risk of developing type 2 diabetes or impaired glucose tolerance.

We think that's pretty convincing stuff!

How do I use the 10 per cent stepping stones if I have a lot of weight to lose?

That's easy. Each time you reach one of your stepping stones, simply recalculate what 10 per cent of your new weight is, and that will give you the next target.

What do I do when I want to stop losing weight?

Easy again. Remember that you can eat a low-GL diet forever, it's so healthy. When you think you've lost enough weight though, you can start to relax a little with your portion sizes. You might choose to eat a little extra bread, for instance, or more nuts. Another good maintenance strategy is what we call the 80/20 rule *(see page 100)* – that's when you watch what you eat most of the time. You might choose to be careful Monday to Friday and relax more at the weekend.

I understand that I may have some lapses, but I'm worried that I'll just give up trying altogether.

Remember, a lapse is just a slip and a relapse is a return to your old ways – the art of a successful lapse is not to let it turn into a relapse. Now, if you've read

this chapter carefully, you should have plenty of
strategies in place already to prevent a relapse, but if
you're still worried about those difficult times we
highly recommend that you join our diet freedom
online club at www.dietfreedom.co.uk, get on the
forums and join in the dialogue. There are so many
people there to support and encourage you that we
can't recommend it highly enough!

Chapter Nine

GET ACTIVE AND FEEL FANTASTIC!

When we think about weight loss we tend to home in on our food or energy intake, but on the other side of the scales is energy expenditure or output.

Even if right now you consider yourself to be an *inactive* person, you might be surprised to know that every second of every day your body is burning energy. The organs in your body need energy to keep working and, wait for it, up to 70 per cent of the energy we use every day is spent keeping our internal organs and muscles ticking over. So what? Well, that means that you only have to affect the remaining 30 per cent and you can make a real difference to your overall energy expenditure. That's why a small change to your day-to-day activity routine really can make all the difference when it comes to losing weight.

When you're active regularly your body doesn't stop burning extra energy as soon as you stop your activity. It carries on for some time after, so you keep getting the benefits for longer. And activity doesn't make you hungry – in fact, being active combined with your low-GL eating plan helps regulate your appetite. Being active increases the amount of fat you lose, and losing fat instead of muscle will make it easier to maintain your results. You don't have to get out of breath and sweaty to be working hard enough to burn fat.

So being active has a whole lot more to offer than simple weight loss. There are real physical and mental health benefits – just look at these!

- ⬇ the risk of heart disease
- ⬇ LDL (bad) cholesterol
- Helps prevent high blood pressure and reduces the tendency for blood pressure to rise as we get older
- Weight-bearing activity helps keep bones strong, protecting against osteoporosis
- ⬆ self-esteem
- ⬆ release of endorphins (feel-good hormones)
- ⬇ risk of depression
- ⬆ sleep quality

All these benefits can be yours no matter what your age or how unfit you are to start with, but if you haven't been active for a while check with your doctor first. They'll be able to advise you about the type and level of activity that's right for you. Start slowly and build up gradually.

Once you've had the okay from the doc, get ready, get set and go, go, go! Choose an activity you'll enjoy (rock-climbing may not be a great idea if you're scared of heights!) and make sure you can afford it. Joining a swanky gym is marvellous, but not if it makes you broke and you never use it. Be realistic about fitting it into your lifestyle – Hollywood stars can do two hours a day at the gym, but they don't have laundry to do, meals to cook and toilets to clean!

Here are some day-to-day examples of great moderate-intensity activities:

- Brisk walking (this is our favourite, so there's more coming up on walking)
- Dancing
- Low-impact aerobics
- Aqua aerobics
- Martial arts
- Jogging
- Cycling
- Swimming
- Tennis

Stepping Out

We told you that we love walking to keep fit and keep the pounds off. There are lots of reasons why it's our top form of activity:

- It's free.
- It's good for you.
- You can do it anywhere.
- You can do it any time.
- You can do it for just a few minutes or for an hour or more.
- It gets us away from these darn computers!

Here's a question for you: in Nigel's clinics, at what life stage do you think most women remember first gaining weight?

Answer: when they stop walking the kids to school. This comes up so many times. The diet didn't change but stopping that 15–20-minute walk there and back everyday was enough to pile on the pounds. Of course, the great message from this is that putting in the extra 15–20-minute walk a couple of times a day will be enough to see those excess pounds melt away. It really does make a difference.

How Much is Enough?

We've talked about starting off gently and building up slowly when it comes to getting active. But we all need to work towards a target to see that we're making progress.

Ideally, 30–40 minutes' brisk walking most days will be enough to keep you fit, and will help most people lose weight when they follow the GL Diet. If you don't want to follow the diet too carefully but think you can definitely get a lot more active, then 50–60 minutes' brisk walking five days a week should still be enough to promote weight loss.

Another good way to measure how much walking you're doing is to wear a pedometer or step counter. A kilometre of walking equates to about 2,000 steps, and studies have shown that some people find counting their steps much more motivating than watching the clock. As far as we're concerned, you should use whichever method you prefer to keep track of your walking, but this table gives you an idea of where you are on the activity front using step counting.

Steps per Day for Different Activity Levels

Steps per day	Activity level	diet freedom says
Under 5,000	Sedentary	Just another 1½ kilometres and you can be up to the next level!
5,000–7,499	Average	Who wants to be average? Come on, go that extra mile!
7,500–9,999	Above average	2 kilometres, that's about 20 minutes' walking at lunchtime, and you've made it to the 10,000 mark!
Over 10,000	Active	Fantastic – you're doing just fine, but of course there's always room for that little bit more!
Over 12,000	Highly active	We take our hats and walking boots off to you – you're a shining example to us all. Well done!

If you think you can do a little more to move up to the next level, these ideas might be just the ticket.

- Walk to work – or part of the way.
- Walk the kids to school.
- Cancel the papers and go collect them yourself.
- Get out of the office at lunchtime for 15 minutes and walk.
- Use the loo on the next floor in the office and take the stairs every time you go.

- Walk the dog or someone else's (or walk a lovely pooch at the local rescue centre!)
- Take a walk after dinner.

How Hard is Hard Enough?

We're always talking about brisk walking, but as with any activity we need it to be of a moderate intensity to really do the business. The 'talk test' is about the most reliable way to make sure you're working hard enough, but not too hard.

The Talk Test

You should be able to maintain a conversation while being active, feel a little warmer and slightly breathless. If you can just chat away as usual, then you can probably go a bit faster, and if you can't talk at all then it's time to slow down because you're overdoing things. And, of course, be sensible. If you think there's any reason why starting to get more active might be a little risky for you, talk to your doctor first.

Is the gym right for me?

Going to the gym can be great but it can also be expensive and even a complete waste of money if you don't use it enough (or at all). Before you sign up to join a gym be sure you can afford the time to go, ask what happens if you need to cancel your membership and also about special off-peak membership if you have free time during the day. In some areas GPs can refer people for exercise free of charge if they are at risk of heart disease – ask about 'exercise on prescription schemes'. If you've got the time and the dedication, then a gym membership can be fantastic.

Is resistance training any good for weight loss?

Resistance training, or using light weights, builds muscle strength and flexibility. Muscle tissue is metabolically active, so it can burn calories. The more muscle tissue you have, the faster your metabolism will be, so yes, adding some hand weights, cans of beans or bottles of water to carry while you walk is great. Remember though, muscle weighs more than fat, so if you start adding resistance to your activity you may actually gain a few pounds even though you are losing inches – it soon catches up though.

Do I need to drink more water while being active?

You sweat to cool yourself down while being active, so yes, you do need to replace that lost fluid. If you're walking briskly for an hour, or if the weather is hot, you may need up to an extra litre of water. It's fine to add a little juice to your water to make it more palatable. Take frequent sips rather than trying to down it in one, and don't wait to feel thirsty before

drinking. Thirst is a delayed reaction to being
dehydrated, so keep well hydrated all the time.

What if I can't get about much?

If it's impossible for you to get up and about, don't
worry. You can still control your weight, but it does
mean it'll be a little harder than for people who can be
active. Some people find swimming is a good option
because the water supports their weight rather than
their joints having to do the work. Chair exercises can
also be really helpful. Your GP's surgery or
physiotherapy department will be able to give you
advice about specific exercises you can do and also
about special activities in your area for people with
reduced mobility.

Activity Research News

Several studies in the US and Finland have shown that physical activity combined with a healthy diet can help prevent type 2 diabetes by up to 58 per cent in high-risk groups like people who are overweight. Research has also taught us that physical activity helps to reduce high blood pressure and high cholesterol and can offer protection against osteoporosis. Of course, the strongest evidence from around the world points to increased activity levels reducing the risk of heart disease and being overweight.

'I feel like shouting from the rooftops. If you'd told me even 10 weeks ago that my life would turn around like this I'd never have believed it.'

Ruth from Lancashire
diet freedom online club member

'I loved the part in The 7-Day GL Diet *about exercise. It's a great approach for someone like me who used to love walking but never has time – 10–15 minutes each day is something I can't say I don't have time for so I'm going to make an honest effort to do that as often as I can.'*

Andie from Essex
diet freedom online club member

'I've been trying to get motivated to exercise for a long time but never seemed to have the energy. Since finding the GL I do! And I've been inspired to try a lot of different activities to see which is my best fit – belly-dancing was fun, Callanetics is great, yoga is perfect, swimming I love – but the easiest to fit into my schedule (I travel a lot so gym memberships are wasted on me) is walking!'

Claire from Florida
diet freedom online club member

'I'm 43 and run my own business. My body has gone haywire since March when I had to curtail the gym visits for a while due to a neck injury. I'm waiting to see a specialist as I seem to be gaining weight, am constantly tired and permanently cold. My GP thinks it may be to do with insulin levels. A friend recommended the GL Diet as a possible solution. Have done it for a week – not really as a diet, just following the principles – and have dropped 7lb and a dress size already. Given that I don't have much to lose, that's about 20–25 per cent of what has to go. I have to say that the family thinks the food is delicious – they've enjoyed the variety.'

Gill from Hertfordshire
diet freedom online club member

'I do think this style of eating puts me much more in control. I'm not always trying to work out ways of having more food, which makes me feel for the first time that I can "keep on keeping up". One pound a week tends to be my weight loss on all diets nowadays but this has been so much easier than other diets. I'm finding the "temptation tamers" helpful and I've written my own list combining the ones that grab me plus a couple of my own. The most useful ones this week have been "I don't eat rubbish any more" and "Just one could be the tip of an iceberg".'

Pam
diet freedom online club member

Chapter Ten

LOW-GL RECIPES

As this is *The GL Diet Made Easy* we decided to make *all* the recipes super fast – so they're all ready in 10 minutes or less! If you have a little more time to spare, you'll love our last book, *The GL Diet Cookbook*.

Food Notes

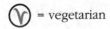 = vegetarian

Milk

You can use any type you fancy. If you're worried about fat, choose skimmed or semi-skimmed. You can also use soya milk or goat's milk if you prefer it to cow's milk.

Cream, Crème Fraîche, Sugar-free Natural Yoghurt

You can interchange these ingredients in most recipes. We love Greek yoghurt because it's creamy and tastes lovely but it's also high in fat (although you can now get low-fat versions), as is cream. If you do use either, take it into account in your overall fat intake for the day. Our favourite lower-fat yoghurt option is bio yoghurt as it's creamier than standard low-fat yoghurts.

Oil

We use olive oil for most things, but in some cases groundnut (peanut) oil is a better choice when cooking at high temperatures as it has a higher 'smoke point'. Look for the organic version.

Natural Low-GL Sweeteners

This is a new and evolving area and unfortunately low-GL natural sweeteners are not widely available at the time of going to press. The best on offer at the time of writing is agave syrup. We recommend that before you get started you visit www.dietfreedom.co.uk where you will find an up-to-date list of our recommended products with stockists for all your low-GL sweetening needs.

Other Ingredients

Most of the ingredients you will need for your new eating plan are very easy to find but for the less commonly known ones we provide a growing list of stockists on our website www.dietfreedom.co.uk

Breakfast

'Seriously, this GL business is so easy. I can't say that the weight is dropping off dramatically but I'm losing steadily as the weeks go by. And I don't feel like I'm on a diet, just making choices without feeling like I'm missing out. My personal recipe discovery is porridge with frozen raspberries stirred in – turns an interesting shade of pink/purple but tastes just like summer pudding. Thanks for all your help!

Sandy from Canterbury

Berry Madness Ⓥ

Ready in: 5 minutes
Serves: 1
1 tbsp blueberries
6 strawberries
2 thin slices Jarlsberg cheese
1 tsp balsamic vinegar (optional)
Freshly ground black pepper

1. Arrange the berries and cheese on a plate.
2. Sprinkle with balsamic vinegar if using.
3. Grind over black pepper.

Fruity Cool Porridge Ⓥ

You can use dried mango, apple, cranberries, pineapple, strawberries or pear, or if you prefer some chopped fresh fruit such as apple, pear, strawberries or raspberries … mmmm!

Ready in: 5 minutes
Serves: 1
30g/3 tbsp/½ cup porridge oats
Your choice of milk (enough to cover – it will absorb)
Handful of dried apricots, chopped
Small handful of any unsalted nuts

1. Soak the porridge oats in milk overnight in the fridge.
2. In the morning sprinkle with the apricots and nuts and eat!

Creamy Coconut Porridge

You can also cook this on the hob in a small pan – it will only take a few minutes longer than the microwave. Try stirring in a teaspoon of unsweetened cocoa for a new breakfast experience!

Ready in: 5 minutes
Serves: 1
30g/½ cup/3 tbsp porridge oats
125ml/½ cup water
125ml/½ cup semi-skimmed milk
1 tbsp desiccated coconut
1 tsp agave syrup
1 tbsp cream

1. Put all the ingredients, except the cream, in a microwaveable bowl, cook for approximately 2 minutes on high and stir briskly.
2. Stir in the cream before serving.

Cinnamon Banana Smoothie

Ready in: 5 minutes

Serves: 1

**1 small, green and yellow, stripy, straight banana
(okay, a bent one will do!)**

2 tsp agave syrup

125ml/½ cup your choice of milk

150g/about ½ cup natural, sugar-free yoghurt

Pinch of cinnamon to taste

1. Slice the banana roughly and place in a blender.
2. Add the rest of the ingredients and blend until smooth.
3. Pour into your favourite glass and serve sprinkled with a little more cinnamon.

Cheesy Bacon Muffins

You can make these in batches and freeze individually wrapped for future 'grab and go' convenience. Just grab one on the way out and it will be defrosted in about 40 minutes. Alternatively, take out of the freezer the night before and leave in the fridge.

You can also cook the muffins in a conventional oven – preheat to 190°C/375°F/Gas Mark 5. Put the mix into a non-stick muffin tin and bake for about 15 minutes.

Ready in: 10 minutes
Serves: 4
30g/2 tbsp olive oil-based spread, melted
2 large free-range eggs
100g/1 cup ground almonds
2 rashers lean, crispy, cooked bacon, cut into pieces
2 tbsp grated cheese such as Parmesan or mature cheddar
1 tsp baking powder
½ tsp paprika (optional), preferably smoked

1. Whisk the melted spread and the egg together.
2. Add the rest of the ingredients and mix thoroughly.
3. Spoon the mix into 4 individual ramekin dishes.
4. Microwave for about 1 minute each, until springy on top. Don't overcook or they'll go rubbery!
5. Delicious hot or cold!

Easy Granola Yog Pot Ⓥ

You can make a large batch of the granola and keep it in the fridge, covered, to use as needed.

Instead of using the microwave, you can cook the granola in a pan on the hob for a couple of minutes until heated through.

Ready in: 5 minutes
Serves: 1
1 dessertspoon olive oil
1 heaped tbsp porridge oats
1 dessertspoon of any chopped or ground nuts
1 tsp agave syrup
1 tbsp Greek yoghurt
Handful of either fresh fruit (strawberries, raspberries, chopped apple or pear) or chopped dried fruits (apricot, apple, mango, strawberries, pear, pineapple or cranberries) or a fine and fruity combo of the above

1. Combine the olive oil, porridge oats, nuts and agave syrup in a microwaveable dish or large ramekin, stirring well.
2. Cook in the microwave on high for 20 seconds or until heated through, taking care not to burn.
3. Remove, stir thoroughly and set aside.
4. In a glass bowl or suitable glass, layer the yoghurt and the fruit alternately and finish off by adding the granola topping.

You can now buy diet freedom flapjacks to crumble over your yoghurt and fruit as a 'quick cheat' granola topping!

Naughty Weekend Breakfast

This is a low-GL take on a naughty treat of a breakfast
– just now and then mind!

Ready in: 10 minutes

Serves: 2

4 rashers lean bacon, grilled

2 large free-range eggs

1 tsp agave syrup

½ tsp vanilla extract

70ml/⅓ cup milk of your choice

2 slices seedy low-GL bread (we use Burgen Soya &
   Linseed)

1 tbsp olive oil-based spread or butter

Shake of cinnamon

1. Grill the bacon on both sides until crispy.
2. Whisk the eggs, agave, vanilla extract and milk together.
3. Cut each slice of bread into 4 triangles, and dip them into the egg mixture until all pieces are well coated and have absorbed some of the mixture (but not so long that they get too soggy)
4. Heat half the spread in the pan and fry the bread until golden.
5. Add the rest of the spread, flip the bread and fry the other side.
6. Arrange on a plate with the bacon, sprinkling a little cinnamon from a shaker over the top

Lunch

'A diet that fits around real life is the only diet that can succeed, I think … a diet that understands I don't have three hours spare every morning to make lunch!'

Daff from Gloucester
diet freedom online club member

Leafy Prawn Salad

Ideal for lunch boxes, this makes a great wrap or 'pitta pocket' as well – use stoneground wholemeal versions of either. You can also experiment with different leaves.

Ready in: 5 minutes

Serves: 1

Approximately 200g fresh, ready-to-eat prawns (you can use frozen but defrost thoroughly first)

1 tbsp mayonnaise

½ tsp paprika

Lots of freshly ground black pepper

1 handful watercress, washed and dried

1 handful baby spinach, washed and dried

1 handful rocket, washed and dried

Lemon wedge to serve

1. Put the prawns into a large bowl with the mayonnaise, paprika and black pepper and mix thoroughly.
2. Chop or rip the leaves.
3. Put the leaves and the prawn mayo in separate containers, and mix before eating with a squeeze of lemon juice.

Fast Onion Soup Ⓥ

Ready in: 10 minutes

Serves: 2

1 tbsp olive oil

2 large onions, sliced finely

1 clove garlic, crushed or chopped or ½ tsp powder or
    purée

100ml dry white wine

750ml/3 cups organic vegetable or meat stock or
    bouillon

1 slice rye bread, toasted

Approximately 100g Gruyère, Jarlsberg or Edam
    cheese, grated

Sprinkling of Worcester sauce

Freshly ground black pepper

Fresh herbs to sprinkle (optional but a lovely addition
    – chives are especially good)

1. Heat the oil in a saucepan, and fry the onions for about 2 minutes.
2. Stir in the garlic and stir for minute or so.
3. Pour in the white wine; let it bubble for about 30 seconds, stirring.
4. Pour in the stock and let the soup boil while you make the croutons.
5. Put half the cheese on the toast, sprinkle with Worcester sauce and grill until melted.
6. Divide the soup between two bowls.
7. Chop the cheesy toast into squares, and put on top of the soup.
8. Sprinkle over the remaining cheese, grind over lots of black pepper and sprinkle with fresh herbs, if using.

Asparagus and Parma Ham Frittata

Fab hot or cold with salad.

Ready in: 10 minutes
Serves: 2
1 tbsp olive oil
1 medium red onion, sliced
6 thin spears of asparagus, woody stems removed
4 large free-range eggs
Freshly ground black pepper
2 pieces Parma ham
4 sun-dried tomatoes (the ones in oil in a jar are best)
1 tbsp grated Parmesan

1. Heat the oil in a non-stick omelette pan.
2. Chop the asparagus into chunks, about 1 inch in size.
3. Add the onion and asparagus and cook for a minute or two.
4. Whisk the eggs together, and pour into the omelette pan.
5. After about a minute, gently stir the eggs to make sure all the veggies are included.
6. Grind over some black pepper.
7. Once the frittata is golden on the bottom, add the strips of Parma ham and sprinkle over the sun-dried tomatoes and Parmesan.
8. Carefully put the pan under a hot grill until cooked through and golden on top.

Tuna Mayonnaise and Watercress Wrap or Pitta Pocket

Ideal as a lunch box!

Ready in: 5 minutes
Serves: 1

1 small can tuna in brine, drained
2 tsp mayonnaise
1 tsp grainy mustard (optional)
Freshly ground black pepper
1 handful watercress, chopped (or rocket or anything leafy – a mix of mustard and cress works well too)
1 small stoneground wholemeal wrap or pitta

1. Mix the tuna, mayonnaise, mustard (if using) and black pepper together and fill the wrap or pitta.
2. Wrap in clingfilm or greaseproof paper if using in a lunch box.

Smoked Salmon Wrap or Pitta Pocket

Ideal as a lunch box!

Ready in: 5 minutes
Serves: 1
1 tbsp half-fat cream cheese
1 tsp creamed horseradish (optional)
1 small stoneground wholemeal wrap or pitta
1 small 'little gem' or iceberg lettuce, sliced thinly
2 pieces smoked salmon
Freshly ground black pepper
Squeeze of fresh lemon

1. Mix the cream cheese and horseradish together and fill your wrap or pitta, layering the lettuce and smoked salmon.
2. Season with black pepper and squeeze over a little lemon juice.
3. Wrap in clingfilm or greaseproof paper if using in a lunch box.

Spicy Chicken and Guacamole Wrap or Pitta Pocket

Ideal as a lunch box! For the chicken you can use a small roasted chicken or turkey breast, sliced chicken, turkey, ham or beef cut into strips. Any other pepper sauce can be used in place of Tabasco, or a pinch of hot chilli powder. Use any herbs/leaves of your choice. You could also use a small chapatti or pancake *(see recipe on page 188)* in place of any of the wraps or pittas.

Ready in: 7 minutes
Serves: 1
1 medium avocado, mashed
2 cherry tomatoes, chopped finely
Juice of ½ lemon
3 dashes Tabasco sauce
1 small stoneground wholemeal wrap or pitta
4–5 slices spicy cooked chicken
1 large handful rocket, basil, coriander or watercress

1. Mix the mashed avocado with the chopped tomatoes, lemon juice and Tabasco and fill your wrap or pitta, adding the chicken and leaves.
2. Wrap tightly in clingfilm or greaseproof paper if using as a lunchbox.

Mighty Mixed Bean Lunch Box Ⓥ

Ready in: 10 minutes

Serves: 1

2 tbsp olive oil

1 small onion, sliced

1 tsp caraway or cumin seeds

**200g/about 1 cup mixed beans (cannellini, haricot,
    chickpeas, pinto beans, kidney beans)**

2 tsp balsamic vinegar

1 handful finely chopped parsley

1 handful watercress, roughly chopped

1. Heat the oil in a small pan, and fry the onion on a medium heat for about 3 minutes.
2. Add the caraway or cumin seeds and stir for a few seconds.
3. Add the beans and cook for another minute, stirring, so the beans all get a good covering.
4. Take off the heat, add the balsamic vinegar and stir.
5. Stir in the parsley and leave to cool.
6. Take the watercress in a separate container, and toss together just before eating.

Energy-boosting Salad

Ready in: 10 minutes

Serves: 2

2 rashers thick-cut lean bacon

2 large free-range eggs

**2 large handfuls rocket, spinach or mixed salad
    leaves**

**1 large handful sprouting seeds (optional, you can use
    more leaves instead)**

**1 heaped tbsp mature cheddar or Parmesan cheese,
    grated**

2 medium tomatoes, cut into quarters

2 tsp balsamic vinegar

1 tbsp olive oil

1 tbsp toasted pumpkin seeds and pine nuts

1. Put the bacon into a small frying pan, without oil, and fry until crispy.
2. Put the eggs in a pan of cold water and boil for 6–7 minutes.
3. Run the eggs under cold water.
4. In the meantime wash and drain the leaves and divide between two plates or large bowls.
5. Put the sprouting seeds on top, if using.
6. Sprinkle over the cheese.
7. Chop up the bacon and scatter over the salad.
8. Peel the eggs, cut into quarters and add to the salad.
9. Put the tomato quarters in the bacon pan, cook for a minute or so, then take off the heat and add the balsamic vinegar and olive oil, stir and allow to warm through.
10. Sprinkle the toasted seeds and pine nuts over the salad.
11. Divide the tomatoes and warm dressing between the two servings, and eat immediately.

Scrambled Egg and Asparagus

Ready in: 10 minutes

Serves: 2

2 generous bunches of asparagus

4 large free-range eggs

1 tbsp olive oil spread

Plenty of freshly ground black pepper

1. Steam or boil the asparagus until just cooked 'al dente'.
2. Whisk the eggs together.
3. Add the olive oil spread to a small pan over a medium heat.
4. Add the eggs and stir until almost cooked.
5. Take off the heat.
6. Drain the asparagus, and arrange with the eggs on a plate.
7. Grind over freshly ground black pepper to taste.
8. Serve immediately.

Easy Homemade Carrot and Coriander Soup Ⓥ

You can also use cooked, fresh carrots or cooked broccoli (add Parmesan instead of coriander) or any leftover cooked vegetables (adding your favourite herbs and spices).

This freezes well if you want to make a big batch and freeze in individual serving sizes.

Ready in: 6 minutes
Serves: 2

1 400g can of baby carrots in water
1 tbsp single cream or crème fraîche
Sprinkle of fresh, chopped coriander or ½ tsp dried

1. Drain the carrots (retain can) and purée in a blender.
2. Add half a can of fresh cold water, the cream or crème fraîche and coriander and stir well to combine.
3. Either place in a microwave-safe bowl, cover and heat for 2 minutes and stir, ensuring it's hot enough *or* pour into a saucepan and heat until boiling, adding more water to thin the soup as required.
4. Stir and serve.

Lacy Egg Soup Ⓥ

For variations, you can use other herbs such as chives, parsley and coriander. Try adding chopped spring onions, chicken or garlic. You can use organic chicken stock instead of vegetable stock.

Ready in: 10 minutes
Serves: 2
600ml organic vegetable stock, bouillon or miso soup
2 large free-range eggs
60g/4 tbsp Parmesan or cheddar cheese, grated
Freshly ground black pepper
Handful fresh basil, finely chopped

1. Bring the stock to a fast boil.
2. Stir in the eggs and cheese, and stir for about 3–4 minutes as it boils.
3. Take off the heat, stir in the pepper and basil.
4. Serve immediately.

Baked Ham and Egg Muffins

You'll need a non-stick muffin pan for this recipe.

Ready in: 10 minutes

Serves: 2

2 large slices of lean ham from the deli counter (not 'plastic' ham!)

4 small free-range eggs

Freshly ground black pepper

1. Cut the ham into 4 pieces and line four of the muffin hollows, making sure there are no gaps.
2. Break an egg into each hollow and bake in a hot oven for about 8 minutes or until the eggs are cooked.
3. Serve hot with toasted rye bread soldiers or cold with a salad and coleslaw.

Easy Homemade Tomato Soup

This freezes well. You can also use any fresh tomatoes – just add water in place of juice. To make a more filling lunch, add a handful of cubed Edam or a sprinkling of mozzarella or Parmesan cheese. A cup of V8 vegetable juice also adds a nice flavour to the soup.

If you want a more spicy soup, add a couple of cloves of crushed or chopped garlic or 1 tsp garlic powder or purée or ½ tsp hot chilli flakes and a few dashes of Worcester sauce.

Ready in: 6 minutes
Serves: 2
1 400g can/2 cups of plum tomatoes, including juice
1 tbsp single cream or crème fraîche
Freshly ground black pepper

1. Liquidize the tomatoes and juice in a large bowl.
2. Stir in the cream or crème fraîche and black pepper.
3. Either place in a microwave-safe bowl, cover and heat for 2 minutes and stir, ensuring it's heated through *or* pour into a saucepan and heat until boiling.
4. Stir and serve.

Warm Pasta, Bean and Tomato Salad Ⓥ

You can add other veggies, such as asparagus, peppers or broccoli. Sun-dried tomatoes can be used instead of fresh ones. Add a couple of chopped anchovies for a bit of a zing!

Ready in: 10 minutes
Serves: 4

200g penne pasta (preferably buckwheat or wholemeal pasta)

3 tbsp olive oil

1 large onion, sliced

1 garlic clove, crushed or grated

2 large tomatoes, quartered

800g/4 cups beans, drained and rinsed (cannellini, haricot, chickpeas, pinto beans)

2 generous handfuls chopped fresh herbs (basil, coriander, chives, parsley, rocket) or dried if you don't have fresh

Juice of 1 lemon

1. Cook the pasta until just cooked or 'al dente', drain and refresh under cold water. Set aside.
2. Heat 1 tbsp olive oil in a large pan, add the onion and fry for a minute.
3. Add the garlic, tomatoes and the rest of the oil, stirring for about 30 seconds (if using dried herbs, add them at this stage).
4. Add the beans and cook for another 5 minutes.
5. Stir in the pasta and herbs.
6. Squeeze over the lemon juice and serve.

Dinner

'I can't believe how much I feel in control of things now after only two weeks of acquainting myself with the whole system. It's truly 'diet freedom'. No counting sins or points or calories, no weighing or calculating ... blessings on the team for thinking up this one!

Karen from Glasgow
diet freedom online club member

Peppery Salad

If you'd like this as a lunch-box or cold option, allow the veggies and dressing to cool down, and keep the dressing separate until you're ready to eat the salad. Any leaves will work in this salad, and you can experiment with your fave veggies too.

Ready in: 10 minutes
Serves: 2
2 handfuls watercress, washed and drained
2 handfuls rocket, washed and drained
2 handfuls baby spinach, washed and drained
4 tomatoes, cut into quarters
2 tbsp olive oil
4 rashers lean bacon, grilled and cut into pieces
1 red pepper, sliced
1 bulb fennel, sliced thinly (optional)
1 small raw beetroot (or cooked), sliced thinly
1 dessertspoon balsamic vinegar
Lots of freshly ground black pepper
40g/approximately 2 tbsp coarsely grated mature
    cheddar

1. Put all the leaves and the tomatoes into a large salad bowl, together with the bacon.
2. Heat one tbsp of the olive oil in a pan. Add the pepper, fennel (if using) and beetroot and fry for 5 minutes or so (if using cooked beetroot, add it at the end).
3. With a slotted spoon, take out the veggies and sprinkle on the salad.
4. Keep the pan on the heat and add 1 tablespoon of olive oil and the balsamic vinegar and black pepper and stir well for about 30 seconds, just until warmed through.
5. Pour over the salad. Toss well, and sprinkle with grated cheese. Serve immediately.

Mediterranean Couscous

Leftovers make a great lunch box the next day – the tastes will have really mingled in! Experiment with other veggies and your fave herb and spice blends.

Ready in: 10 minutes

Serves: 4

150g/¾ cup couscous, cooked as per packet instructions and drained

1 courgette, sliced into chunky rounds

1 aubergine, cut into rounds then quarters

1 red pepper, cut into strips (about 1cm wide)

1 tbsp olive oil

1 clove garlic, crushed or chopped, or ½ tsp dried or purée

1 tsp harissa paste (or other warm paste/sauce)

Plenty of freshly ground black pepper

1 generous handful fresh mint and parsley, finely chopped (or use dried)

1. Preheat your grill to hot.
2. Put the veggies into a bowl with the olive oil, garlic, harissa and black pepper and toss.
3. Put the bowl to one side for later and lay the veggies on the grill.
4. Cook until turning golden then turn over and cook on the other side.
5. Put the cooked couscous into the bowl the veggies were tossed in.
6. Add the cooked veggies and the chopped herbs, toss well.
7. Serve warm or cold.

Seared Strips of Beef with 'Cabbaghetti'

We love our 'cabbaghetti'. It tastes really good – yes, really! You may even fool the kids into thinking it's something other than the dreaded cabbage.

Ready in: 10 minutes
Serves: 2
1 small cabbage, washed and shredded
1 tbsp olive oil
2 lean beef steaks, cut into strips
Freshly ground black pepper
1 tbsp soy sauce
1 dessertspoon Parmesan

1. Steam or boil and drain the shredded cabbage thoroughly or cook in the microwave with a tbsp of water and drain well.
2. Heat the oil in a pan and fry the steak with the black pepper for 2–3 minutes until cooked through, stirring.
3. Add the soy sauce, heat through and stir.
4. Divide the cabbaghetti onto 2 serving plates.
5. Drizzle over a little extra olive oil and sprinkling of Parmesan.
6. Spoon the steak and sauce over the cabbaghetti and serve.

Tagliatelle with Spinach and Mushrooms Ⓥ

Ready in: 10 minutes

Serves: 2

1 tbsp olive oil

125g button mushrooms, washed and sliced

1 clove garlic, crushed or chopped or ½ tsp dried or purée

200g fresh egg tagliatelle or any fresh pasta (we also love buckwheat pasta – it's very filling and yummy!)

1 bag of baby spinach leaves, washed

2 tbsp crème fraîche, natural sugar-free yoghurt or single cream

50g chopped walnuts

1. In a large pan fry the sliced mushrooms and garlic in the olive oil until golden brown.
2. In the meantime cook the pasta in a pan of boiling water for about 3 minutes or until just cooked, and drain thoroughly.
3. Add the cooked pasta to the pan of mushrooms and garlic.
4. Now add the spinach and cream/yoghurt/crème fraîche and stir together over a low heat until the spinach has wilted.
5. Divide onto 2 serving plates and sprinkle with the chopped walnuts.

Perfect 'Baked' Pasta ⓥ

You can experiment with other veggies and herbs. If
you prefer, you can use buckwheat pasta instead of
tortellini, and half-and-half pasta and beans (such as
butter beans).

Ready in: 10 minutes

Serves: 4

1 tbsp olive oil

1 large onion, finely chopped

1 fennel bulb, finely chopped (optional)

4 cloves garlic, crushed or grated

800g/4 cups chopped tomatoes (usually 2 cans)

4 dashes Worcester sauce

4 dashes Tabasco sauce

400g fresh tortellini filled with cheese, tomato,
    spinach or meat

1 big handful fresh basil, chopped

75g/5 tbsp mature cheddar, coarsely grated

25g/2 tbsp Parmesan cheese, finely grated

1. Heat the olive oil in a large pan, and add the onion and fennel (if using).
2. Add the garlic and fry for about 2 minutes.
3. Add the chopped tomatoes, Worcester sauce and Tabasco.
4. Leave to bubble gently over a low heat for a couple of minutes.
5. In the meantime, boil the pasta as per the packet instructions until 'al dente' then drain well.
6. Set your grill to a high heat.
7. Transfer the tortellini to an ovenproof serving dish, sprinkle with basil (reserve a bit to garnish) and pour over the sauce.
8. Sprinkle over the two cheeses and put under the grill until bubbling and golden brown.
9. Serve immediately with a big crisp salad.

Pancakes Ⓥ

Pancakes are fast to make and freeze well. You can make up a batch and then just take them out of the freezer and pop them in a warm pan or microwave to defrost when you fancy a pancake or a speedy wrap! You can use the pancakes cold as an alternative to the wraps and pitta breads *(see pages 162–4)*.

Ready in: 10 minutes
Makes 6 large or 10 small pancakes
100g/1 cup buckwheat flour (this has a lower GL than wheat flour – you can also use spelt or stoneground wholemeal flour, but bear in mind they will have a higher GL)
1 large free-range egg
250ml/1 cup your choice of milk
125ml/½ cup water
1 tbsp Greek yoghurt
Groundnut (peanut) oil (has a higher 'smoke point' than olive oil – but you can use olive oil if needs be)

1. Whisk the flour, egg and milk together until you get a smooth paste.
2. Whisk in the water and the yoghurt until you have a smooth batter.
3. Heat a teaspoon of oil in a small non-stick pan – just enough to cover the base.
4. Add enough batter to just cover the bottom of the pan and swirl the batter around until the base is thinly covered.
5. Cook on one side until golden. Flip gently as they are quite delicate at this stage. Repeat until all the batter has been used.
6. Use immediately or allow to cool and then separate with greaseproof paper, place in a plastic bag and freeze.

Ideas for Pancake Fillings

- Stuff with smoked salmon, asparagus and scrambled eggs.
- Add in 1–2 tbsp chopped fresh herbs to the batter. Fresh basil is gorgeous!
- Stir-fry your favourite veggies and wrap them in a warmed pancake with a sprinkle of grated cheese, or pour over a hot tomato- or cheese-based sauce.
- Stir-fry some chicken or turkey strips with bean sprouts and soy sauce.
- Put a line of shredded lettuce down the middle, top with cooked spicy chicken pieces, sprinkle over some grated cheese, roll up and pop under the grill for a couple of minutes for a 'melt'.
- Use to make 'cannelloni' by filling with 200g cooked and drained spinach mixed with 200g ricotta cheese, a teaspoon of grated nutmeg and lots of black pepper – roll up tightly and place in a microwaveable dish, top with a spicy tomato sauce and thin slices of mozzarella cheese and cook on high for a few minutes until heated through (or bake in a hot oven for 15–20 minutes).

New Potato, Salmon and Dill Combo

Ready in: 10 minutes

Serves: 2

1 tbsp olive oil

2 large boneless salmon fillets, diced

**1 can of baby new potatoes, drained and halved
(enough for two)**

8 cherry tomatoes, halved or 4 tomatoes, quartered

1 dessertspoon fresh chopped dill or 1 tsp dried

**2 tbsp natural sugar-free yoghurt, single cream or
crème fraîche**

Freshly ground black pepper

1. Heat the oil gently in a large frying pan over a
   medium heat and fry all the ingredients except for
   the yoghurt/cream/crème fraîche.
2. When the salmon is cooked through, add the
   yoghurt/cream/crème fraîche to the pan with
   1 tbsp of water or enough to make a sauce
   consistency.
3. Season with black pepper, and continue to cook
   until heated through and serve with lots of green
   veggies or a crunchy salad.

Courgette and New Potato Fritters

These are lovely cold as well, and will be a good addition to a lunch box. Keep them in the fridge, covered, for a couple of days for 'snack attack' time too. They're also delicious as a side dish to curry instead of rice or bread.

You can add 1–2 tsp curry powder to the mix, or try using other veggies – carrots, sweet potatoes, parsnips and celeriac all work well.

Ready in: 10 minutes
Serves: 4 (makes about 16)
1 medium courgette, coarsely grated
1 large onion, grated
Freshly ground black pepper
1 tsp cumin seeds (optional)
**2 tbsp gram (besan) flour (or you can try spelt or
    buckwheat flour)**
1 large free-range egg
**1 tbsp organic vegetable oil or groundnut (peanut) oil
    for cooking**

1. Mix the grated veggies in a large bowl and stir in the pepper, cumin (if using) and gram flour.
2. Beat the egg and stir into the veggie mixture.
3. Heat the oil in a pan over a high heat and add 1 tbsp of the mix at a time – flatten the mix out in the pan so it's about 5cm round and 1cm thick.
4. Turn gently once golden, and drain on kitchen paper once cooked.
5. Serve with a large salad or other low-GL veggies of your choice.

Sweet Potato and Turkey Omelette

Ready in: 10 minutes

Serves: 2

1 medium sweet potato, washed and chopped into
    small chunks

1 tbsp olive oil

2 shallots or 1 small onion, finely chopped

4 slices cooked turkey, cut into strips

4 large free-range eggs

Freshly ground black pepper

Generous handful of chives, washed and chopped
    (fresh will taste best but you can stir in a tsp of
    dried instead)

100g/approximately ¾ cup mature cheddar, grated

1. Boil or microwave the sweet potato until just cooked and drain well.
2. Heat the oil in a non-stick omelette pan.
3. Add the shallots/onion and sweet potatoes and fry for about a minute until golden, then add the turkey.
4. Whisk the eggs together in a bowl, stir in plenty of black pepper and the chives.
5. Pour the egg mix into the pan and allow to cook for a minute, then gently push it around a bit to make sure the turkey and veggies are well covered.
6. When the underside is golden, sprinkle the cheese on top and put under a hot grill until the top is golden and the omelette is cooked through.
7. Serve immediately with a big crispy 'n' crunchy green salad.

Speedy Burgers

Use whichever herbs you like for this recipe. You can also try minced chicken, turkey or beef instead of the pork. If you prefer, you can roll the mix into meatballs before cooking.

To use cold for lunch box wraps or pitta pockets, chop some fresh herbs like mint and oregano into some yoghurt or cream cheese and add to the wrap/pitta with crisp lettuce and chopped tomatoes.

Ready in: 10 minutes

Serves: 4

1 medium onion, roughly chopped

4 cloves garlic, peeled

1 handful fresh parsley, roughly chopped or 1 tsp dried

2 tsp freshly ground black pepper

450g/1lb lean minced pork

1 tbsp fine oatmeal

1 tbsp olive oil

1. Put the onion, garlic, parsley and pepper into your blender, and blitz until finely chopped.
2. Add the pork mince and oatmeal and 'pulse' until mixed well.
3. Pat into burgers – 4 large or 8 smaller.
4. Heat the oil in a pan and put the burgers on to cook, flipping them to brown both sides.
5. Serve hot with 'cabbaghetti' *(see page 182)*, a large green salad or a tomato-based pasta sauce.

Turkey Sweet 'n' Spicy Stir-fry

Ready in: 10 minutes

Serves: 4

4 turkey breasts, sliced thinly

1 tbsp agave

½ tsp hot chilli powder

2 tsp fresh grated ginger or 1 tsp dried

1 tbsp olive oil or groundnut (peanut) oil

1 large onion, sliced

2 cloves garlic, crushed or chopped

2 red peppers, sliced

2 sticks of celery, diced

100g sugar snaps or mangetouts

1 cabbage, shredded

1 tbsp soy sauce

1 tsp toasted sesame oil (optional)

1. Toss the sliced turkey in the agave, chilli and ginger.
2. Heat the oil in a wok or large frying pan.
3. Add the turkey and stir-fry until golden on all sides.
4. Add the onion and stir-fry for a few seconds.
5. Stir in the garlic, peppers, celery and sugar snaps/mangetout and stir-fry for another couple of minutes.
6. Once you're sure the turkey is cooked, add the cabbage and the soy sauce, stirring vigorously for another couple of minutes.
7. Take off the heat, drizzle over the sesame oil, toss and serve.

Fast 'n' Fab Fish Fingers with Mash 'n' Peas

Very popular with the kids – they won't know the mash isn't potato! Try adding fresh mint to the water when boiling the peas. Also great with vegetable chips – cut your favourite root veggies (such as carrots, parsnips, swede, sweet potato) into wedges and roast like oven chips.

Ready in: 10 minutes
Serves: 4

1 large cauliflower, cut into about 8 pieces
450g/3 cups frozen peas
2 tbsp olive oil or groundnut (peanut) oil
1 large free-range egg
4 tbsp fine oatmeal
Freshly ground black pepper
2 large fillets of boneless white fish (cod, plaice, hoki etc.)
1 tsp creamed horseradish
1 tsp olive oil-based spread
Lemon wedges to serve

1. Steam, boil or microwave the cauliflower until tender and set aside to drain really well.
2. Boil or microwave the peas – these only take a couple of minutes – drain and keep warm.
3. Heat the oil in a large pan.
4. Whisk the egg.
5. Put the oatmeal on a plate and mix in some black pepper.
6. Cut the fish fillets into 'fingers' and dip first in the egg then roll in the oatmeal and fry for a couple of minutes until cooked. Keep warm in the oven.
7. Mash the cauliflower (as you would potato), mixing in the creamed horseradish, spread and black pepper and serve up with lemon wedges.

Lemon Chicken with Fresh Basil Salad

Ready in: 10 minutes

Serves: 2

2 large cooked skinless and boneless chicken breasts, sliced

410g can/2 cups cannellini beans, drained and rinsed

2 tbsp roasted red peppers, drained (you can buy them in oil in jars from supermarkets)

1 tbsp extra virgin olive oil

1 tbsp lemon juice

Freshly ground black pepper

Handful of fresh basil leaves, washed or ½ tsp of dried (fresh is so much nicer though!)

1. In a large bowl combine the sliced chicken breasts, beans and red peppers.
2. Whisk the olive oil, lemon juice and black pepper together (if using dried basil add here) and add to the other ingredients in the bowl.
3. Add whole fresh basil leaves, toss together and serve.

Tomato Tuna

Ready in: 10 minutes
Serves: 2

1 tbsp olive oil
1 medium onion, chopped
1 tsp cumin seeds
1 tsp caraway seeds
½ tsp hot chilli flakes
2 tuna steaks
410g can/2 cups chopped tomatoes, drained
Juice of 1 lemon
Freshly ground black pepper
Handful fresh chopped coriander to serve
Lemon wedges to serve

1. Heat the oil in a large pan.
2. Add the onion and the spices and stir-fry for about 30 seconds.
3. Add the tuna and fry gently on both sides.
4. When the tuna is cooked through, add the chopped tomatoes, lemon juice and black pepper. Simmer for a couple of minutes.
5. Sprinkle with coriander and serve with lemon wedges, salad or low-GL veggies.

Desserts

'This isn't a breakthrough "lose 10 pounds in a week" miracle diet. It's the way we should eat. It respects our general health as well as our shape. It's more a way of eating which will get you to where you should be, but getting there is very enjoyable and easy. I love food and cooking. This has improved my skills and repertoire. Today is appropriate to give this tribute to diet freedom as I bought myself my long-promised pair of white boot-cut jeans in a comfy size 10 this afternoon, and I looked at the bikinis too!'

Estella from Newcastle
diet freedom online club member

Dark Chocolate-dipped Strawberries

Only for special occasions – no, the dog's birthday doesn't count. Goldfish? Don't even go there!

You can also melt the chocolate in the microwave, but be very careful not to burn it. Break into squares and put in for 10 seconds at a time. Keep stirring each time until melted.

Ready in: 10 minutes
Serves: 2

12 strawberries, washed with stalks left on
100g chocolate, 70 per cent cocoa content (we love
Green & Blacks Cook's Chocolate)

1. Melt the chocolate gently in a bowl over a pan of hot water.
2. Lay out a large piece of greaseproof paper on a baking tray.
3. Quickly dip each strawberry into the bowl of melted chocolate until it is covered from the bottom to the middle, and put onto the greaseproof paper.
4. Repeat until you've used up all the strawberries and chocolate!
5. Allow to cool in the fridge, and then gently peel off the greaseproof paper.

Fig and Ricotta Pots ⓥ

You can use Greek yoghurt or crème fraîche in place of the ricotta. Try strawberries or other berries or fruits in place of the figs.

Ready in: 5 minutes
Serves: 2
2 fresh figs
Few sprigs of mint
4 tbsp ricotta cheese
Handful of slivered almonds, toasted
1 dessertspoon agave syrup

1. Cut the figs into quarters and arrange in the bottom of two dessert bowls (glass ones look very pretty!).
2. Chop most of the mint finely, reserving two sprigs for decoration, and sprinkle over the figs.
3. Spoon over the ricotta cheese, dividing it equally between the two bowls.
4. Sprinkle with the toasted almonds (you can toast them yourself in a dry pan for a couple of minutes).
5. Drizzle over the agave and decorate with a mint sprig in each bowl.

Yoghurt Sponge Pud Ⓥ

Ready in: 8 minutes

Serves: 2

1 dessertspoon agave syrup

60g ground almonds

30g natural, sugar-free yoghurt

2 tsp olive oil or olive oil-based spread

1 large free-range egg

½ tsp baking powder

1 tsp natural vanilla extract (we love the Nielsen-
  Massey vanilla extract – it really makes a
  difference to the taste)

1. Place all the ingredients in a microwave-proof pudding bowl and whisk or beat together until thoroughly mixed.
2. Cook on high in the microwave for 2–3 minutes or until risen and springy on top. Don't overcook or you'll end up with a rubbery pud … and we can't have that peeps, can we now?

Fruit 'n' Cheese Ⓥ

'Dessert' doesn't need to be complicated and loaded with sugar. This fruit 'n' cheese platter is a great option. Fruit should be firm and just ripe as the GL will be lower. Use your fave fruit and cheeses.

Ready in: 5 minutes
Serves: 4
150g Jarlsberg cheese
150g firm goat's cheese
1 pear
1 apple
Handful of strawberries
Handful of grapes

1. Slice the cheese thinly and arrange on a plate.
2. Slice the pear and apple and arrange on the same plate.
3. Put the strawberries and grapes in the middle.
4. Put into the middle of the table and graze as you chat!

Berry Lemon Mousse Ⓥ

You can use other fruits in place of the summer berries.

Ready in: 7 minutes

Serves: 4

Zest of 3 lemons (keep a few 'curls' of zest for decoration or use a sprig of mint)

Juice of 2 lemons

220g/1 cup ricotta cheese

3 tbsp agave syrup

250ml/1 cup whipping cream

8 tbsp summer fruits (fresh or frozen and defrosted)

1. Mix the lemon zest, juice, ricotta and agave syrup.
2. Whip the cream until it forms soft peaks and then gently mix with the ricotta and lemon.
3. Divide the summer fruits between four dessert bowls (nice glass ones!).
4. Spoon the lemon mousse over the top of the fruit.

Creamy Chocolate Pancakes

We love the chocolate sauce in this recipe – it's fabulous! We also love those mini whisks you can get now – they're perfect for whisking small quantities like this *(see ww.dietfreedom.co.uk for where to buy)*.

You can add chopped strawberries or other summer berries or try shop-bought sugar-free fruit purée. Fresh lemon or orange juice or pureed raspberries or strawberries can be used on the top instead of the chocolate sauce.

Ready in: 5 minutes

Serves: 4

2 tbsp sugar-free cocoa

1 tbsp boiling water

2 tbsp agave syrup

4 buckwheat pancakes *(see recipe on page 188)*

2 tbsp thick Greek yoghurt or mascarpone cheese

1. Whisk the cocoa, hot water and agave together to make a divine chocolate sauce.
2. Heat the pancakes in a dry pan or microwave if using from frozen so they are slightly warmed.
3. Blob the yoghurt down the middle of each pancake.
4. Drizzle with a little chocolate sauce.
5. Fold each pancake in half and drizzle a little more of the chocolate sauce over the folded pancake.
6. Serve to many ooooooh's of delight!

Sweet Vanilla Peaches Ⓥ

This will also work with figs, plums and a warm berry compote.

Ready in: 10 minutes
Serves: 4

4 peaches
1 tbsp agave syrup
1 tbsp ricotta cheese
1 tsp vanilla extract
Sprigs of mint

1. Preheat your grill to hot.
2. Cut the peaches in half, remove the stones and slice.
3. Arrange in an ovenproof dish and drizzle with agave syrup.
4. Put under the grill for about 5 minutes.
5. Mix the ricotta cheese and vanilla extract together.
6. Spoon the peaches into individual bowls and top with the vanilla ricotta.
7. Decorate with sprigs of mint.

50 'Easy' Snacks

While in weight-loss mode you can have up to two snacks a day – mid-morning and mid-afternoon. Try not to go for more than four hours without eating something to help keep your blood sugars stable. Choose from the following list and make at least one of your daily snacks fruit or vegetable based.

Fruit Snacks

Make sure the fruit is still firm and only just ripe – as fruit ripens the GL increases.

1. 1 apple
2. 1 pear
3. 1 tangerine
4. 1 satsuma
5. 1 orange
6. 1 small semi-ripe banana (still green striped)
7. 1 apricot
8. 1 peach
9. 1 plum
10. 1 small handful of grapes (green or red)
11. 1 small handful of cherries
12. 1 small handful of blackberries
13. 1 small handful of strawberries
14. 1 small handful of raspberries

15. 1 small handful of blueberries
16. 1 small handful of pitted prunes
17. Half a small grapefruit
18. 1 kiwi
19. 1 small slice of watermelon
20. Quarter of a small melon
21. Half a papaya (pawpaw)
22. 1 Ugli fruit
23. 1 small handful of dried apricots
24. 1 small handful of dried blueberries
25. 1 small handful of dried apple
26. 1 small handful of dried cranberries (make sure they're sugar-free)

Other Snacks

27. Matchbox-sized piece of any cheese
28. 1 mini Edam cheese
29. 1 cream cheese triangle
30. 2 squares of dark chocolate (at least 70 per cent cocoa)
31. 1 small handful of seeds or unsalted nuts or a mixture (Don't overeat either seeds or nuts – they're very calorie dense and it's easy to have too many. If you aren't losing weight, cut them out until you reach your target weight.)
32. 1 small handful pitted or stuffed olives
33. 3 cherry tomatoes
34. 1 small handful unsweetened popcorn

35. 1 oat cake with olive oil spread or cream cheese
36. 1 Ryvita (or similar rye crispbread) with olive oil-based spread or cream cheese
37. 1 small teacup of sugar-free vegetable soup (not potato or pasta based) – tomato, asparagus, broccoli or onion are good choices
38. 1 small teacup of tomato or vegetable juice
39. 1 small sugar-free yoghurt drink
40. 1 dessertspoon of houmous with vegetable dippers
41. 1 dessertspoon of cheese and chive dip with vegetable dippers
42. 1 dessertspoon of guacamole dip with vegetable dippers
43. 1 dessertspoon of tomato salsa dip with vegetable dippers
44. 1 dessertspoon of red pepper pâté with vegetable dippers
45. 1 dessertspoon of smoked salmon pâté with vegetable dippers
46. 1 dessertspoon of tuna pâté with vegetable dippers
47. 1 dessertspoon of coleslaw with vegetable dippers
48. Half a small avocado with a squeeze of lemon juice and a drizzle of balsamic vinegar and olive oil
49. Half a hard-boiled egg spread with cream cheese or pâté
50. Handful of washed, sweet baby carrots – you can buy them in bags from the supermarket pre-washed. A great snack!

Vegetable dippers = peppers, cucumber, carrots or celery
cut into chunky strips

Pâtés = red pepper, mushroom, smoked salmon, tuna,
mackerel, crab or any other fish – either shop-bought or
homemade

Dips = cream cheese, cheese and chive, tomato salsa,
guacamole, tzatziki, coleslaw, houmous or garlic –
either shop-bought or homemade

Chapter Eleven

A–Z OF LOW-GL FOODS

Here's the A–Z list of healthy, low-GL foods to base your meals on (not a packet of biscuits in sight!). Please read through Chapter 4 first – this will give you our top tips for achieving that overall nutritional balance which makes the GL Diet so healthy.

More new foods are being tested for their GI/GL all the time, including many branded products. We aim to give you the most up-to-date information available, so if you would like to keep yourself up to speed with newly tested low-GL foods, you can join our diet freedom online club at www.dietfreedom.co.uk.

If the food is normally eaten cooked we give you the cooked weight of our recommended portion, unless otherwise stated. All foods listed have a low GL of 10 or less. If foods haven't been tested yet, but we assume they'll have a low GL based on similar foods, we've included them (you'll see NT, which stands for 'not tested', in the GL column). Foods that contain either no carbohydrate or only a minimal amount are listed as 0 in the GL column. The 0 foods will have no glycaemic impact. So the bottom line is that if a food is on the list it's fine to eat as part of a low-GL diet! Enjoy …

A

	Recommended portion size	GL
Agave syrup	10g	2
Anchovies*	120–50g	0
Apple juice	125ml	6
Arrabiata sauce	2–3 tbsp	NT
Artichoke	80g	0
Asparagus	80g	0
Aubergine (eggplant)	80g	0
Avocado	80g	0
Avocado, mint and lime dressing	1 tbsp	NT

B

	Recommended portion size	GL
Baked beans	80g	4
Balti sauce	2–3 tbsp	NT
Banana	60g	6 (yellow and green)
Banana	60g	3 (green – under-ripe)
Banana (small)	60g	7 (ripe)
Bean sprouts	80g	NT
Beef	75–120g	0
Beetroot	80g	4
Blackberries	120g	0
Black-eyed beans	80g	5
Black pepper sauce	2–3 tbsp	NT
Blueberries	120g	0

	Recommended portion size	GL
Blueberry juice	125ml	7
Bolognese sauce	2–3 tbsp	NT
Bran sticks (sugar free)	30g	NT
Bread and crackers – although we give the approximate GL for 30g of bread/crackers below, a good guideline would be no more than one slice of bread per day for women (or two crackers) and two for men (or four crackers) while trying to lose weight. You won't find all these breads in your local supermarket, but they're becoming more widely available. Try your local health food shop. If in doubt, go for the darkest, grainiest bread you can find. It'll have more fibre, be less processed and have a lower GL than the highly refined white-flour breads. Gluten-free breads tend to have a moderate GL as they are often based on corn.		
Broad beans	80g	5
Broccoli	80g	0
Brown rice	75g	9
Brussels sprouts	80g	0
Buckwheat kasha (boiled, cooked weight)	100g	10
Bulgur wheat (boiled, cooked weight)	100g	8
Butter	20g	0

	Recommended portion size	GL
Butter beans	80g	3
C		
Cabbage	80g	0
Caesar dressing	1 tbsp	NT
Carrot juice	125ml	5
Carrots	80g	2
Cashew nuts	50g	3
Cauliflower	80g	0
Caviar	1 tbsp	0
Celeriac	80g	0
Celery	80g	0
Chana dal	80g	2
Chasseur sauce	2–3 tbsp	NT
Cheese – all types	50–75g	0
Cheese and chive dip	1 tbsp	NT
Cheese and onion dip	1 tbsp	NT
Cheese sauce	2–3 tbsp	NT
Cherries	120g	3
Chicken	100–150g	0
Chickpeas	80g	4
Chicory	80g	0
Chilli dressing	1 tbsp	NT
Chocolate – choose chocolate with at least 70 per cent cocoa. A few squares as a snack are a great healthy choice!		

	Recommended portion size	GL
Coffee is fine but be aware that some coffee-bar chains add sugary syrups to their coffees which will make them high GL – ask for plain coffee or a cappuccino.		
Coleslaw	1 tbsp	0
Collard greens	80g	0
Courgettes (zucchini)	80g	0
Couscous (cooked weight)	100g	7
Cranberry juice	125ml	8
Cream	1 tbsp	NT
Crème fraîche	1 tbsp	NT
Cucumber	80g	0
D		
Dark Swiss rye bread	30g	9
Diet drinks	1 can/small bottle	NT
Dips – a tablespoon would be a sensible portion. Check for added sugars if buying ready-made versions.		
Dressings – a tablespoon would be a sensible portion. Check for added sugars if buying ready-made versions.		
Dried apple	60g	10
Dried apricot	60g	9
Dried peach	60g	8

	Recommended portion size	GL
Dried prunes	60g	6
Dried fruits – All dried berries such as strawberries, raspberries, blueberries and cranberries are fine. Look for sugar-free versions – cranberries often have sugar added. Dried apple, apricot and peach have all been tested as low GL for 60g. Pineapple and mango haven't been tested but should be low to moderate. Dried pear has been tested as 12 GL for 60g so is moderate. Raisins, however, have a high GL of 27 for 60g as do sultanas at 25 GL for 60g, so use sparingly if at all. Dried figs and dried dates also have a moderate to high GL score.		
Duck	100–150g	0
E		
Eggs (free range or organic)	1	0
Endive	80g	0
F		
Falafel	100g	NT
Fettuccine, egg-based pasta	100g	10
Figs (fresh)	120g	NT

	Recommended portion size	GL
Fish – Approximate uncooked portion sizes are white fish 150–200g, all oily fish/tuna and salmon 120g–150g, shellfish 120–150g. Aim to eat three portions of fish per week, with at least one being oily fish.		
Flaxseeds	50g	NT
Forestière sauce	2–4 tbsp	NT
French dressing	1 tbsp	NT
Fructose	10g	2
Fruit – The vast majority of fruits have a low GL. We've given the GL for a 120g portion but you don't need to weigh them – just guesstimate. Berries are very low GL and a brilliant choice. Stick to firm fruit – if it's soft and over-ripe the GL will be higher.		
Fruit juice – Choose juices that contain 100 per cent fruit and aren't made from concentrate, preferably with bits of fruit or pulp which means more fibre and a lower GL. Limit to 125ml maximum per day and mix with water to make a longer drink.		
Fruit tea	unlimited	NT

	Recommended portion size	GL
G		
Game	100–150g	0
Garlic is great and so good for you! Include fresh garlic in your cooking.		
Garlic and herb dip	1 tbsp	NT
Goat's milk (maximum total milk per day ½ pint or 284ml)	125ml	NT
Grapefruit	120g	1–3
Grapefruit juice	125ml	4–6
Grapes – black	120g	10
Grapes – green	120g	8
Guacamole	1 tbsp	NT
H		
Haricot/navy beans	80g	6
Hazelnuts	50g	NT
Hemp seeds	50g	NT
Herbal tea	unlimited	NT
Herbs and spices – use generously to add lots of flavour and interest to your food for both taste and decoration. If you can't be bothered fiddling with fresh herbs (you can freeze them or buy frozen) use dried instead.		
Herrings*	120–150g	0
Honey	25g	10

	Recommended portion size	GL
Honey and mustard dressing	1 tbsp	NT
Houmous	1 tbsp	<1
I		
Ice cream	50g	3–8 (variable)
J		
Jalfrezi sauce	2–3 tbsp	NT
Jam, reduced sugar	30g	5
K		
Kale	80g	0
Kidney	75–120g	0
Kidney beans	80g	5
Kippers*	120–150g	0
Kiwis	120g	6
Kohlrabi	80g	0
Korma sauce	2–3 tbsp	NT
L		
Lamb	75–120g	0
Leeks	80g	0
Lemons	1	0
Lentils	80g	3
Lettuce (all types)	80g	0
Lima beans	80g	5

	Recommended portion size	GL
Limes	1	0
Linseeds	50g	NT
Liver	75–120g	0
M		
Macadamia nuts	50g	NT
Mackerel*	120–150g	0
Madeira sauce	2–3 tbsp	NT
Madras sauce	2–3 tbsp	NT
Mandarins	120g	NT
Mangetout	80g	0
Mangoes	120g	8
Maple syrup	25g	9
Mayonnaise	1 tbsp	NT
Meat – Choose fresh, lean cuts of meat over processed ones as they often have added sugars. Buy organic where possible. An approximate portion guide (uncooked) is red meat 75–120g, poultry and game 100–150g. Try to keep to no more than three portions of red meat per week.		
Meat alternatives – Soya and Quorn (vegetable micro-protein) are good low-GL choices.		
Melons	120g	4

	Recommended portion size	GL
Milk, cow's (maximum total milk per day ½ pint or 284ml)	125ml	2
Muesli – Look for sugar-free versions or make your own	30g	7–16 (variable)
Mung bean noodles, dried	100g	8
Mung beans	80g	5
Mushroom sauce	2–3 tbsp	NT
Mushrooms	80g	0
N		
Napoletana sauce	2–3 tbsp	NT
Nectarines	120g	NT
Nuts are very nutritious but are loaded with calories so stick to no more than a small handful of unsalted nuts a day. If you don't lose weight cut them out until you reach your target weight.		
O		
Oat bran (raw)	10g	3
Oat bran and honey bread	30g	7
Oatcakes	30g	8
Okra	80g	0
Olive oil	1 tbsp	0
Olive oil spread	20g	0
Olives	80g	0

	Recommended portion size	GL
Onions	80g	0
Orange juice	125ml	5
Oranges	120g	5
Ostrich	100–150g	0
P		
Papaya/pawpaw	120g	9–10
Parsnips	80g	8

	Recommended portion size	GL
Pasta and noodles – Try and keep these to smaller portions as an accompaniment rather than the largest part of the meal. Make sure you cook them 'al dente' (firm to the bite) as the longer they're boiled the higher the GL rises! Gluten-free corn pasta has a moderate GL. We've given the GL for 100g cooked weight. Both our own experience and feedback from our fabulous GL dieters has told us that the amount of pasta and noodles you can eat and still lose weight varies significantly from one person to the next – so start with smaller amounts and see how it affects you. Mixing beans and pulses with pasta and noodles will enable you to have a bigger portion and lower the GL of the overall meal. All weights refer to cooked weight unless otherwise stated.		
Pâtés – Fish pâté is a great way to get some of your oily fish quota and a healthier choice than the meat versions which can be very high in fat.		
Peaches	120g	5
Peanuts	50g	1

	Recommended portion size	GL
Pearl barley (cooked weight)	100g	5
Pears	120g	4
Peas	80g	3
Peas (marrowfat)	80g	4
Peas (split yellow)	80g	3
Pecans	50g	NT
Peppers	80g	0
Pesto sauce	2–3 tbsp	NT
Pilchards*	120–150g	0
Pine nuts	50g	NT
Pineapple juice	125ml	8
Pineapples	120g	7
Pinto beans	80g	5
Pistachio nuts	50g	NT
Plums	120g	5
Pomegranate juice	125ml	12 (use sparingly)
Popcorn (plain, microwaved)	20g	8
Pork	75–120g	0
Porridge oats (steel cut, cooked in water)	30g (dry weight)	9
Potatoes (baby new)	80g	6
Prunes (pitted)	60g	10
Pumpernickel bread	30g	5
Pumpkin	80g	3
Pumpkin seeds	50g	NT
Puttanesca sauce	2–3 tbsp	NT

	Recommended portion size	GL
Q		
Quinoa	100g	9
This is the latest test result for boiled quinoa (results have been variable in the past).	(dry weight)	
R		
Radicchio	80g	0
Radishes	80g	0
Raspberries	120g	0
Ravioli	100g	8
Red pepper dressing	1 tbsp	NT
Red wine and herb sauce	2–3 tbsp	NT
Rhubarb	120g	0
Rice – Long-grain rice and basmati rice still have a GL over 10, even for 75g, so use brown rice or wild rice instead.		
Rice bran, extruded (cooked weight)	30g	3
Rice noodles	100g	10
Roasted vegetable sauce	2–3 tbsp	NT
Runner beans	80g	0
Rye, whole	30g (dry weight)	8
Rye crackers	30g	10
S		
Salmon* (canned or fresh)	120–150g	0

	Recommended portion size	GL
Sardines*	120–150g	0
Sauces – A sensible portion would be 2–3 tablespoons per person. When choosing ready-made sauces, dips and dressings look for ones without added sugar, glucose/glucose syrup or dextrose – better still make your own with fresh ingredients so you know exactly what's in it!		
Sauerkraut	80g	0
Sausages – Choose 90 per cent meat plus	75–120g	0
Scallions (green onions)	80g	0
Semolina (steamed)	100g	4
Sheep's milk (maximum total milk ½ pint or 284ml per day)	125ml	NT
Shellfish	120–150g	0
Soba (buckwheat) noodles	100g	NT
Soups – Most are low GL. Choose the most natural ones you can find. Fresh cartons are often the best choice GL wise – check tins as they sometimes contain hydrogenated/trans fats. Look for ones which include low-GL ingredients and skip the potato- and pasta-based ones. Good soup choices would be tomato,		

	Recommended portion size	GL
tomato and basil/herb, asparagus, leek, broccoli, vegetable, lentil, pea, French onion – in fact, any low-GL vegetable as per the vegetable list.		
Sour cream	1 tbsp	0
Sour cream and chive dip	1 tbsp	NT
Sourdough rye bread	30g	6
Soya (meat alternative)	100–150g	NT
Soya and linseed bread (Burgen)	30g	3
Soya beans	80g	<1
Soya milk (maximum total milk ½ pint or 284ml per day)	125ml	2
Soya yoghurt	100g	6
Spaghetti, white	100g	10
Spaghetti, wholemeal	100g	9
Spelt hasn't been tested yet so use sparingly for now.		
Spelt multigrain bread	30g	7
Spinach	80g	0
Spinach and ricotta or nutmeg sauce	2–3 tbsp	NT
Spring onions (scallions)	80g	0
Squash (all)	80g	0
Strawberries	120g	1
Sunflower and barley bread	30g	6
Sunflower seeds	50g	NT
Swede	80g	7

	Recommended portion size	GL
Sweet pepper sauce	2–3 tbsp	NT
Sweet potatoes	80g	9
Sweetcorn	80g	9
Sweeteners – Artificial sweeteners such as aspartame, sucralose and saccharin are generally low GL. Some people find them useful but we prefer to use small amounts of agave syrup as a natural low-GL alternative to sugar. We don't recommend polyols such as xylitol or maltitol as they can cause gastrointestinal distress in some people – their GI/GL values vary and they can cause immediate laxative effects! Some companies use polyols as sweeteners in their low-carb products and use the term 'net carbs', but this is controversial and confusing, especially as the effects of polyols vary from one to the next. Until specific low-carb products are tested for their GI/GL and shown to have little effect on your blood sugars we wouldn't recommend them. Visit www.dietfreedom.co.uk for up-to-date advice on sweeteners and stockists.		
Swiss chard	80g	0

	Recommended portion size	GL
T		
Tabbouleh	50g	NT
Tangerines	120g	NT
Tarragon sauce	2–3 tbsp	NT
Tea (black/green)	unlimited	NT
Tikka masala sauce	2–3 tbsp	NT
Tinned fruits are fine but make sure they're in their own juice rather than sugary syrups. Check the label for added sugar.		
Tinned vegetables – Check there's no sugar added.		
Tomato and basil dressing	1 tbsp	NT
Tomato and basil sauce	2–3 tbsp	NT
Tomato and mascarpone sauce	2–3 tbsp	NT
Tomato and roasted onion dressing	1 tbsp	NT
Tomato juice	125ml	2
Tomato salsa	1 tbsp	NT
Tomatoes	80g	0
Tortellini, cheese	100g	6
Tuna*	120–150g	0
Turkey	100–150g	0
Turnips	80g	0
Tzatziki	1 tbsp	NT

	Recommended portion size	GL
U		
Ugli fruit	120g	NT
V		
Vegetables – Try to eat a rainbow of coloured vegetables every day to get a good variety of antioxidants, vitamins and minerals – at least three portions per day if you can. The weights given apply to cooked vegetables but you may want to eat some of them raw.		
Vinaigrette dressing	1 tbsp	NT
W		
Walnuts	50g	NT
Watercress	80g	0
Watercress sauce	2–3 tbsp	NT
Watermelon	120g	4
Wheat, whole	30g (dry weight)	8
White fish	150–200g	0
White wine sauce	2–3 tbsp	NT
Wholegrain bread	30g	7
Wholemeal pitta bread (look for 'stoneground' as it'll be less processed)	30g	10
Wholemeal rye bread (look for 'stoneground', as above)	30g	8

	Recommended portion size	GL
Wild rice	75g	8
Y		
Yams	80g	7
Yoghurt	200g	2–4
Yoghurt and mint dressing	1 tbsp	NT
Yoghurt drinks (sugar free)	1 standard size	NT

Chapter Twelve

BURNING QUESTIONS ABOUT GL

Can I eat bananas?

Yes, stick with a small one though as they're high in sugar. Under-ripe ones have a much lower GL – so greener rather than brown!

Which types of potatoes have the lowest GL?

You can find the GL of potatoes in the food lists. The potatoes with the lowest GL are baby new potatoes, either fresh or tinned, and sweet potatoes. Large white baking potatoes have a higher GL, as do French fries!

What are the best low-GL breads currently available?

You can buy Burgen bread (it's Australian) in most UK supermarkets. It's a brown, sliced loaf made from soya and linseeds and has a lower GL than most bread. Try keeping it in the freezer and taking out a slice as you need it so that you aren't tempted to eat too much of it. Pumpernickel or rye bread also has a low GL as it's grainy, dense and not over-processed. Generally, the darker whole-grain breads are the best choice GL wise. You may prefer to eat oatcakes or rye crispbreads instead of bread, so see which suits you best.

What is the best natural low-GL sweetener available?

This is a new and evolving area and unfortunately low-GL natural sweeteners are not widely available at the time of going to press. The best on offer at the time of writing is agave syrup, although it is expensive. Visit www.dietfreedom.co.uk before you get started where you will find an up-to-date list of our recommended products with stockists for all your low-GL sweetening needs.

Are nuts allowed on a low-GL diet?

Yes, but only a small handful a day. Although nuts are low GL they are very easy to overeat and very calorie dense! Monitor how they affect your weight loss – some people seem to stall when eating nuts and others don't. Stick to the natural, unsalted ones and see how you go. Almonds are particularly good as they help lower cholesterol!

Does adding lemon juice and/or vinegar to foods lower their GL?

Yes, anything acidic such as lemon juice or vinegar lowers the GL of a food or meal, so get squeezing! You can make some lovely dressings with lemon juice, olive oil and herbs.

Can I eat butter?

We recommend that you use olive oil, an olive oil-based spread or a small amount of butter. All have a zero GL. Avoid the low-fat spreads that contain hydrogenated/trans fats, now being banned in many countries as they've been linked with heart disease and cancer. Check the label.

Why haven't all foods been tested for their GL?

Testing has to be done in a controlled laboratory setting. It includes taking blood samples from a group of volunteers and comparing their blood glucose levels after eating the test food, and again after eating the same amount of available carbohydrates from glucose. Testing is therefore both expensive and time consuming to carry out. To begin with scientists just tested basic carbohydrate foods but now many food manufacturers are starting to have their own products tested and to show their glycaemic response on packaging. We think this is a good move and will help give us more information about the food we eat and how our bodies react to it. More foods are being tested all the time. We keep an updated list of tested foods on the members section of our website www.dietfreedom.co.uk.

Why don't I need to count calories on the GL Diet?

By reducing the 'overall' GL of our daily diets we can help prevent fat storage. Providing we stick to the few quantity recommendations on certain foods and eat until we're satisfied rather than 'stuffed' there's no need to count calories, and anyway it's boring. You obviously can't eat loads of calorie-dense foods like nuts and cream every day and expect to lose weight, but since glycaemic testing started we now know that calories are only part of the equation, and simply reducing them is not the weight-loss Holy Grail it promised to be.

Do I have to count GL points?

No, definitely not. We have a lot of ex-points and calorie counters who now love the freedom of low GL. Although it takes a while to kick the counting habit, the diet freedom that ensues is just brilliant to behold. Lowering the overall GL of your diet by using the advice and food lists in this book will get you on the road to eating healthily and losing weight at the same time – a double whammy. That really is all you need, along with a bit of a boost to your activity level (*see Chapter 9*). Eating a low-GL diet will help regulate your appetite naturally and prevent those blood sugar lows after eating high-GL foods that have you heading for the biscuit tin or rooting through the cupboards for something sugary!

For all those control freaks out there, you can count your daily GL score if you really want to by using the A–Z food list in Chapter 11. Aim to eat no more than 80 GL per day if you want to lose weight. If you're overweight you're probably consuming a high-GL diet of 120 GL plus per day.

Is this a low-fat diet?

No. A lot of research has been done on fats, and most experts now agree that it isn't the overall quantity that counts but the quality and type of fat we eat. Kick the hydrogenated/trans fats into touch, keep saturated fats to a minimum and bring out the olive oil. We recommend using olive oil and olive oil-based spreads to increase your intake of these good monounsaturated fats that are heart healthy. The information we give on portion sizes will help keep your total fat intake at a healthy level.

How much weight can I expect to lose and how quickly?

Losing weight too quickly is a recipe for disaster and increases the likelihood of unhealthy yo-yoing. A

weight loss of around 2 pounds per week is a
sensible, safe rate. Some people lose more if they
have a lot of weight to lose to begin with. The GL Diet
is based on sound science and healthy-eating
principles and isn't a quick-fix fad. In fact, it isn't a
diet but a permanent life choice. Your weight loss will
depend on many factors, including your age, exercise
level, genes, general health, metabolism, medications
you're taking and the total amount of weight you have
to lose.

Do I have to weigh myself every day?

This can be a bit negative to be honest; especially for
women as their water retention varies so much
depending on cyclical hormonal changes. How you
wish to keep track of your weight loss, though, is your
choice. Weighing once a week or every two weeks is
preferable, and don't forget to measure specific areas
before you start and every week after that. You'll be
amazed at your rate of inch loss. For other ideas for
monitoring your success, see pages 120–24.

What affects the GL of food/food products?

Apart from the composition of the ingredients, other
factors that influence the GL are:

- the type and degree of processing
- ingredient interactions; which is why testing products is important – some ingredients can slow down or speed up the absorption of others
- the ripeness of some fruits and vegetables
- adding acidity such as lemon/lime juice or vinegar – this can lower the GL of a food
- fibre content – some high-fibre ingredients slow down gastric emptying (a stage in digestion), which also reduces the GL

How does a low-GL diet help control hunger?

Low-glycaemic foods are digested and absorbed more slowly than high-glycaemic foods. This means they take longer to reach the lower part of the small intestine, which in turn makes us feel full and keeps us feeling fuller for longer. Stress hormones such as cortisol and adrenalin are released when glucose levels go up and down after a high-glycaemic meal – both of which stimulate appetite.

Can an underactive thyroid problem make it harder to lose weight?

This can often be the case as a shortage of thyroid hormone can reduce your temperature and your metabolic rate. This in turn leads to fatigue and a lack of energy so that being active can prove really difficult. If you think you may have a thyroid problem, have a look

at www.thyroiduk.org, an informative charity website
set up for sufferers which gives a symptom checklist.

My partner and I have different activity levels. He's very active and I'm not. How do I manage our different dietary needs?

The GL Diet is a perfectly healthy diet for someone
who's very active. The only adaptations you may wish
to consider are to make low-GL carbohydrate portions
larger and more frequent than for someone less active.
Your partner may find it useful to keep a few higher-
GL snacks to use after training in order to replace lost
glycogen stores. Slow carbs will provide long-lasting
energy for everyday needs and the vast majority of
sports, but higher-GL faster carbs may be useful if
short sustained bursts of energy are needed, such as
for sprint training or power lifting. Clearly your partner
will have higher general energy requirements than
you, but these can be met by more frequent meals and
larger portion sizes of low- to moderate-GL foods
rather than overindulging in high-energy, high-GL
snacks. There's a lot of research going on in the area
of sports nutrition which we're keeping an eye on.

I have a wheat intolerance. Can I still use the 'free from' products on the GL Diet?

The 'free from' ranges in many supermarkets often
contain high-GL ingredients, including sugar, high-

fructose corn syrup, corn and rice flours. If your intolerance is to wheat only and not gluten then you should be able to eat 100 per cent rye bread and spelt flour bread. You can also buy buckwheat (it isn't wheat but is from the rhubarb family) or chickpea pasta as an alternative. Corn-based pasta has a moderate GL. You can also find buckwheat noodles or mung bean noodles in Chinese supermarkets and some everyday supermarkets – these have a low to moderate GL. When using these pastas and breads, do still apply the portion guidelines as per the A–Z food lists in Chapter 11. Please also check the label on anything you buy to make sure there's no hidden wheat in the ingredients, and always follow your doctor's advice regarding any kind of intolerance or allergy that may affect your health.

'I've suspected for a while that wheat and potatoes are a dietary problem for me. Since cutting them both right down and using the GL Diet I've had no problem with cravings, bloating or what had previously been diagnosed as IBS. I've also lost weight without much effort at all and have much more energy, which means I'm motivated to exercise as well. It's made a big difference to me!'

Jane from Cardiff

Is it safe to follow the GL Diet when you are pregnant?

It wouldn't be a good idea to try and lose weight during your pregnancy, but the GL Diet is a perfectly healthy diet to support your pregnancy and maintain a healthy weight throughout. Normal weight gain during a pregnancy is around 10–12kg (22–26½lb). After you've had your baby you shouldn't try to lose weight whilst breastfeeding.

Is this a low-carb diet?

The GL Diet takes into account both the quality and the quantity of the carbohydrates we eat – so it's the best of both worlds. We've combined this with general healthy-eating principles so it's also balanced, varied and not restrictive.

How come some people can eat anything without gaining weight?

We all know people who eat loads, including all the wrong things, and *still* never seem to put on any weight. They've been blessed with a genetically high metabolic rate, which means they'll always be slim. The vast majority of us, sadly, have a slower metabolism and a genetic predisposition to store fat for a rainy day. This means that, had we lived hundreds of years ago, we would have survived in times of famine!

Can I eat desserts?

Try to avoid desserts whilst in weight loss mode as most are high GL and loaded with sugar. If, however you really miss having something sweet after dinner you can have either a fruit salad or a diet freedom 'guilt free' treat such as a brownie, carrot cake or flapjack and just eat a little less to compensate during the day.

How do I know which foods are low GL?

Don't panic! We've worked it all out so you don't have to. In our books we provide you with simple lists of low-GL foods (*see Chapter 11*) and specially developed low-GL recipes (*see Chapter 10*). As part of our online membership service we also provide an updated list of tested low-GL foods as new generic and branded foods are tested around the world – see www.dietfreedom.co.uk.

Are there any supportive products?

You don't need to buy *any* products to follow the a low-GL diet, but for those of you who (like us) are time poor, we have painstakingly developed a range of 'natural', low-GL, no sugar added, GM-free, wheat-free, 'guilt-free' treats that contain only non-hydrogenated fat to keep you (and us) on the low-GL track when temptation strikes! So far we have flapjacks, brownies and carrot cake. You can keep up to date with our product launches and stockists on our website www.dietfreedom.co.uk.

How many meals and snacks can I have in a day? Does it work like a points system?

You should aim for three low-GL meals and two low-GL snacks per day to make sure you don't go for more than four hours without eating. This will help keep your blood sugars balanced and ensure you don't feel hungry. There isn't a set points/counting system – it's a way of eating for life. However, if you would like a daily guideline, try to keep your daily GL score to 80 or below when in weight-loss mode (*see the A–Z food lists in Chapter 11*). Obviously the higher your activity level the higher the GL score per day you can get away with and still lose weight.

Can I still eat chocolate?

Yes, just substitute dark chocolate (at least 70 per cent cocoa), which has only a small amount of sugar in it compared to milk chocolate. You'll find it hard to eat more than a couple of squares as it's very rich. If you fancy a cocoa/chocolate sauce as a treat, unsweetened cocoa mixed with a small amount of agave syrup is one of our favourites.

How much tea and coffee can I drink?

A moderate amount of caffeine (from two to three cups of tea or coffee a day) is perfectly fine. If you do want to use decaffeinated coffee, the best choice is coffee that's had the caffeine removed by water rather than chemical processing. This process 'flushes' the caffeine out of the beans prior to grinding. Water-processed decaf coffee is generally a little more expensive than the chemically treated versions. You can find it in health food stores.

Where can I get more advice?

Visit our website www.dietfreedom.co.uk, where you can become a member of the diet freedom online club. You'll meet lots of fellow diet freedomers who enjoy a good chat in our busy forums and in the process support each other, very successfully, to reach their goals. We provide an interactive 'Ask the dietician' service, one-to-one consultations by phone and face to face, newsletters, and an extensive recipe database plus lots more. We never cease to be amazed by the intelligence, insight and information (not to mention humour) that emanates from the forums and would highly recommend you pay them a visit. All three of us post in the forums regularly and offer help and support wherever we can. You'll also find a regularly updated '♥ shopping' section and archive with details of new, tasty and exciting low-GL foods,

interesting activities and just plain gorgeous things!
The website will also keep you up to speed with what
we're up to at diet freedom HQ. We're currently very
busy extending (and tasting – oh yes!) our 'guilt-free'
products – so very exciting times! If you are interested
in the diet freedom 'guilt free' treat range and would
like to see them in a store near you do email us – you
may also like to volunteer as a tester at the same time!
Email guiltfree@dietfreedom.co.uk

I have diabetes. Can I follow the diet?

Yes. A low-GL diet as part of a healthy lifestyle can
help control your diabetes and reduce your risk of
long-term diabetes-related complications (*see page 24
for further details*).

Is a low-GL diet suitable for vegetarians and vegans?

Vegetarians can follow the same healthy low-GL
principles as meat eaters, choosing foods from each
of the major food groups: high protein sources,
cereals and grains, dairy products (or soya
substitutes), vegetables and fruits. Obviously the more
restrictive the diet, the more difficult it becomes to
ensure all the body's nutritional requirements are
being met.

I have PCOS and have been told this diet will help control my symptoms. Can you explain why?

Polycystic ovary syndrome (PCOS) affects up to 10 per cent of women, although many don't realize they're suffering from the condition. We've had some excellent results in easing and reversing symptoms of PCOS with a low-GL diet (*see page 29 for details, and our website www.dietfreedom.co.uk for testimonials*).

Will this diet help balance my moods, especially during PMS?

A low-GL diet helps control the release of the hormone insulin. Many women find a low-GL diet helps improve hormonally driven symptoms associated with premenstrual syndrome, polycystic ovary syndrome and the menopause. So, stick to the GL Diet and monitor the reduction of your symptoms (*see page 29 for more details*).

I have IBS – can I still follow the plan?

Yes. There's no special diet to follow to treat IBS – just a healthy balanced diet, and that's exactly what the GL Diet is.

Irritable bowel syndrome (IBS) is a chronic disorder, which causes the bowel or gut to be oversensitive. The main symptoms are:

- Abdominal pain and tenderness, especially on the left side or across the lower abdomen
- Bloating and fullness of wind
- Constipation
- Diarrhoea
- Alternating between constipation and diarrhoea
- A sensation of having to rush to the toilet
- Pain, relieved by opening the bowels
- Lethargy
- Headaches

The disorder commonly affects people between the ages of 20 and 30 and is twice as common in women as in men. In general, up to one in five adults suffers from IBS and 60 per cent of patients see a specialist gastroenterologist.

Nobody really knows what causes IBS. Sometimes the colon is seen to be in a state of unusual activity, contracting and relaxing in an abnormally rapid way, hence the pain and discomfort. This is also the reason why so many sufferers can hear bowel noises – loud rumblings and squeaking caused by gases being propelled through the intestines. The colon muscle of a person with IBS begins to spasm after only mild stimulation and is more sensitive than usual. It's also well known that IBS could be a mind-body disease, meaning that symptoms may be worse when under psychological stress or even when the body is

physically stressed, such as by an infection or
exhaustion.

There are a number of treatments and approaches.
It's usually a case of experimentation to find which
suits you best. As always, talk through any treatments
beforehand with your health professional.

- Antispasmodics (reduce the spasm in the wall of the
  bowel)
- Peppermint oil
- Painkillers
- Mild antidepressants
- Probiotics

Other treatments or approaches:

- Self-help and support groups
- Cognitive behavioural therapy
- Hypnotherapy
- Relaxation exercises (yoga and Pilates)

Can my whole family eat low GL?
The whole family can benefit from following a low-GL
diet, whether they want to lose weight or just stay
healthy. We have strived to make sure that all the
important aspects of healthy eating have been
incorporated into the GL Diet so that it can be a diet
for life and for everyone.

A low-GL diet means we give our bodies a steady drip feed of energy and can keep going for longer, just like a car with a full tank of fuel on a long journey. A healthy, balanced, low-GL diet can help children to concentrate and avoid the sugar highs and lows associated with bad behaviour.

Will my doctor know about GL?

Many doctors are now aware of GI and GL in relation to diet. We have many members who are either GPs or specialists and follow the diet themselves and recommend it to their patients. If your doctor isn't familiar with GL, you can pass on our contact details or direct them to our website at www.dietfreedom.co.uk and we'll be happy to discuss any aspect of the diet with them.

What about alcohol?

When you consume alcohol your body uses it as a preferential fuel so you have to burn it off before you burn any fat. Remembering that you are delaying fat-burning whenever you indulge in alcohol may be enough to put you off!

You'll lose weight far more easily and quickly if you don't drink alcohol. If you must indulge, red wine is probably the best choice as at least it does appear to offer some health benefits, but only an occasional glass! Think of alcohol as empty calories (no protein, vitamins or minerals) you can do without (guess our popularity has just sunk to an all-time low now … ah well!).

I only eat ready-meals. How can the GL Diet possibly work for me?

Very easily. Looking a little more closely at the labels will help you decide which ready-meals are the best to choose. The shorter the list of ingredients, the better – if you understand what most of them are, and they sound like basic foods, that's great! Look out for things like sugar, glucose and high-fructose corn syrups in the ingredients – the higher on the list the more it contains.

Avoid anything with rice, pasta or potatoes included – you can add other low-GL foods yourself. It's possible to get lots of variations in fish and meat dishes with sauces. The following sauces all provide good accompaniments to beef, pork, chicken, fish or vegetarian meat alternatives:

- Cheese
- Mushroom
- Any tomato-based sauce
- Spinach and ricotta
- Red pepper
- Black pepper
- White or red wine
- Tarragon

- Forestière
- Pesto
- Watercress
- Chasseur
- Asparagus
- Spinach and nutmeg

Add some speedy low-GL vegetables to your meal – there are plenty of ready-prepared vegetable packs that will microwave in minutes. Pre-prepared salad selections are even speedier!

Can I stop the diet once I reach my target weight or size?

If you return to your old eating habits that made you put weight on in the first place then you will obviously start gaining the weight again. The simple answer would be to stick to the GL principles but increase your portion sizes of some foods.

By the time you've reached your desired size and shape you'll not only see the benefits of eating a low-GL diet, but you'll also feel far better health wise with increased energy levels, clearer skin and less irritating health problems such as flu, colds and sore throats.

Another major benefit of balancing blood sugar levels is increased emotional stability with no sugar-induced mood swings and depression. So, just stick with your low-GL principles and remember that eating

low-GL foods is not just about losing weight but
retaining and improving your health as well.

- You could have low-GL desserts after your evening
  meal.
- A handful of nuts a day would be a good healthy
  addition.
- You may also wish to increase your intake of bread to
  maintain your weight rather than continue losing, but
  stick with the low-GL breads.

There's one major problem with following the GL Diet
we feel we should warn you about (and your partners,
come to think of it). We've had numerous complaints
about it in the past – you may well find it necessary to
go out and buy yourself a whole new wardrobe of
clothes but c'est la vie!

Need More Help and Support?

Our website (www.dietfreedom.co.uk) is an online resource for all things GL and health related. You can join our online **diet freedom online club** and gain access to the following exclusive services:

'Ask the Dietician'

Personal and confidential responses to your questions direct to your inbox, plus a database of FAQs. We keep our members up to speed on all things GL, including the latest tested foods.

Forums

Our lively forums provide a great support network with members from all over the world. It's fun, friendly and inclusive – we as authors post regularly. It's our inspiration, and the feedback we receive is of huge importance to us.

One to ones

If you need a bit more emotional support with your weight issues we provide either 'face-to-face' or phone consultations with our team of qualified, registered dieticians. Members receive a discount on all consultations.

Food Lists

Members have access to our low-GL food list and portion guide, which is constantly updated with newly tested foods.

Recipe Database

We add more recipes each week and are building the largest database of low-GL recipes in the world!

Newsletter

Our bi-monthly members' newsletter keeps you up to speed on all things GL with success stories, latest health research, competitions, goodies and lots of gossip of course!

Recommended Suppliers

Although you can easily follow a low-GL diet without buying special foods, you can visit the '♥ shopping' section of www.dietfreedom.co.uk for a list of stockists for any of the recommended low-GL alternative ingredients mentioned that may be difficult to find on the high street. For example:

- Agave syrup
- Buckwheat flour
- Buckwheat pasta
- Range of 70 per cent plus cocoa dark chocolate
- Gram flour
- Oatmeal
- Spelt flour

Recommended Reading

Denby, Nigel, Michelucci, Tina and Pyner, Deborah,
    The GL Diet Cookbook, HarperThorsons, 2006

Denby, Nigel, Michelucci, Tina and Pyner, Deborah,
    The 7-Day GL Diet, HarperThorsons, 2005

Denby, Nigel, Michelucci, Tina and Pyner, Deborah,
    The GL Diet, John Blake, 2004

Denby, Nigel, Baic, Sue, *GL for Dummies*, Wiley, 2006

Denby, Nigel, Baic, Sue, *Nutrition for Dummies*,
    Wiley, 2005

References

Chapter 3: This Diet is Seriously Good for Your Health

Obesity

'Low-glycaemic diets and health: implications for obesity.' Livesey, G. *Proc Nutr Soc*. 2005 Feb; 64(1):105–13.

'Effects of an ad libitum low-glycaemic load diet on cardiovascular disease risk factors in obese young adults.' Ebbeling, C.B., Leidig, M.M., Sinclair, K.B., Seger-Shippee, L.G., Feldman, H.A., Ludwig, D.S. *Am J Clin Nutr*. 2005 May; 81(5):976–82.

'Effects of a low-glycaemic load diet on resting energy expenditure and heart disease risk factors during weight loss.' Pereira, M.A., Swain, J., Goldfine, A.B., Rifai, N., Ludwig, D.S. *JAMA*. 2004 Nov 24; 292(20):2482–90.

Children

'Low glycaemic index breakfasts and reduced food intake in preadolescent children.' Warren, J.M., Henry, C.J., Simonite, V. *Pediatrics.* 2003 Nov; 112(5):e414.

'A reduced-glycaemic load diet in the treatment of adolescent obesity.' Ebbeling, C.B., Leidig, M.M., Sinclair, K.B., Hangen, J.P., Ludwig, D.S. *Arch Pediatr Adolesc Med.* 2003 Aug; 157(8):773–9.

Cancer

'Glycaemic index, glycaemic load and risk of endometrial cancer: a prospective cohort study.' Silvera, S.A. *Public Health Nutr.* 2005 Oct; 8(7):912–9.

'Incidence of colorectal cancer in relation to glycaemic index and load in a cohort of women.' McCarl, M., Harnack, L., Limburg, P.J., Anderson, K.E., Folsom, A.R. *Cancer Epidemiol Biomarkers Prev.* 2006 May; 15(5):892–6.

'Consumption of sweet foods and breast cancer risk in Italy.' Tavani, A., Giordano, L., Gallus, S., Talamini, R., Franceschi, S., Giacosa, A., Montella, M., La Vecchia, C. *Ann Oncol.* 2006 Feb; 17(2):341–5. Epub 2005 Oct 25.

'Dietary glycemic load and risk of colorectal cancer in the Women's Health Study.' Higginbotham, S., Zhang, Z.F., Lee, I.M., Cook, N.R., Giovannucci, E., Buring, J.E., Liu, S; Women's Health Study. *J Natl Cancer Inst.* 2004 Feb 4; 96(3):229–33.

'Dietary glycemic load, carbohydrate, sugar, and colorectal cancer risk in men and women.' Michaud, D.S., Fuchs, C.S., Liu, S., Willett, W.C., Colditz, G.A., Giovannucci, E. *Cancer Epidemiol Biomarkers Prev.* 2005 Jan; 14(1):138–47.

'Dietary carbohydrates and breast cancer risk: a prospective study of the roles of overall glycemic index and glycemic load.' Silvera, S.A., Jain, M., Howe, G.R., Miller, A.B., Rohan, T.E. *Int J Cancer.* 2005 Apr 20; 114(4):653–8.

'Glycaemic index, glycaemic load and risk of prostate cancer.' Augustin, L.S., Galeone, C., Dal Maso, L., Pelucchi, C., Ramazzotti, V., Jenkins, D.J., Montella, M., Talamini, R., Negri, E., Franceschi, S., La Vecchia, C. *Int J Cancer.* 2004 Nov 10; 112(3):446–50.

'Glycaemic index, glycaemic load and risk of gastric cancer.' Augustin, L.S., Gallus, S., Negri, E., La Vecchia, C. *Ann Oncol.* 2004 Apr; 15(4):581–4.

'Dietary glycaemic load and breast cancer risk in the Women's Health Study.' Higginbotham, S., Zhang, Z.F., Lee, I.M., Cook, N.R., Buring, J.E., Liu, S. *Cancer Epidemiol Biomarkers Prev.* 2004 Jan; 13(1):65–70.

'Glycaemic index, glycaemic load, and incidence of endometrial cancer: the Iowa women's health study.' Folsom, A.R., Demissie, Z., Harnack, L; Iowa Women's Health Study. *Nutr Cancer.* 2003; 46(2):119–24.

'Glycaemic index and glycaemic load in endometrial cancer.' Augustin, L.S., Gallus, S., Bosetti, C., Levi, F., Negri, E., Franceschi, S., Dal Maso, L., Jenkins, D.J., Kendall, C.W., La Vecchia, C. *Int J Cancer.* 2003 Jun 20; 105(3):404–7.

Coronary Heart Disease

'Effects of an ad libitum low-glycaemic load diet on cardiovascular disease risk factors in obese young adults.' Ebbeling, C.B., Leidig, M.M., Sinclair, K.B., Seger-Shippee, L.G., Feldman, H.A., Ludwig, D.S. *Am J Clin Nutr.* 2005 May; 81(5):976–82

'Effects of a low-glycaemic load diet on resting energy expenditure and heart disease risk factors during weight loss.' Pereira, M.A., Swain, J., Goldfine, A.B., Rifai, N., Ludwig, D.S. *JAMA.* 2004 Nov 24; 292(20):2482–90.

Diet Freedom Online Club Members' Comments

'While browsing a women's website and chatting to others about GI someone recommended the GL Diet to me. I bought the book and found it very easy to read – it all made such perfect sense and I thought this is the one that's really going to work for me! I've really got into the swing of this eating plan now and eat loads more fruit and veg than I used to, drink a lot more water, not so much red meat but lots more fish, which I love anyway and is in abundance here in Brittany. I feel so much better for it and the best thing is it's the only plan I can remember trying (believe me, I've tried them all in the last 30 years!) that I can imagine following for life.'

Louise from Brittany, France

'I love the current book and can't wait to buy the new one! Am considering selling all the other diet books I own. I doubt I'll find anyone interested in them here on the diet freedom forums though. Well done all.'

Hils from Hampshire

'I've tried most diets, I think! Most were a total failure even after a promising start. Others were almost over before they began because of the major lifestyle change that had to occur. The GL Diet isn't like that – it was very easy to understand, and with a few comparatively minor adjustments I started to lose weight steadily. The GL fits with my very hectic lifestyle and I certainly have much more energy for my 4am starts at the flower market (I work for a florist). I even have enough energy to continue throughout the day and into evening client meetings too! I've lost 2 stone 4 pounds in just nine months and am now at my "longed for" target weight, and stay here pretty effortlessly. I'm thrilled with the GL, and delighted to say at long last that I won't ever need another diet!'

Caroline from London

'My copy of your new book has just arrived and I am inspired! It's very informative, readable and motivational. I'm back on the straight and narrow and feel great! Thanks for another great book!'

Lucy from Plymouth

'Thank you so much for the book. It really is liberating. Over the past couple of weeks I've felt energized with get-up-and-go each morning. I'm feeling healthy and losing weight, which makes me want to exercise, a no-no before. Great book, so easy to read and understand, with positive affirmations that make absolute common sense. Very thoughtful and a definite plus to me. Keep up the good work. Nothing else has worked so I was a bit sceptical – yet my looking and feeling good says it all.'

Stella
Chrysalis Coaching Company

'Bought the GL Diet book last week and have read it cover to cover. OMG! How much sense does it make! I do generally eat a healthy balanced diet. However, I had no idea that the type of carbs eaten had such an influence on how I felt and it has totally explained why the cravings occurred.

'On Monday I made a conscious effort to change the type of foods that I ate and so far so good – I haven't had a single craving for any type of food. I no longer "need" that biscuit with my coffee or the packet of crisps as an afternoon snack. I just hope I'll continue to feel this way with my new eating lifestyle.

'I must say even though I've only been following the GL plan for a week I've already started to notice a difference with my energy levels. I no longer feel tired in the afternoon, whereas before I would normally be yawning my head off by 3 o'clock! Thanks again.'

Kim from Scotland

Index

Index of Recipes

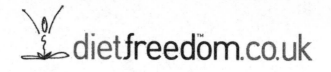
dietfreedom.co.uk

Join our Online Members' Club

Ask the dietician
Confidential answers to your questions direct to your inbox with searchable database.

Low-GL food lists
Constantly updated list of low-GL foods with GL ratings and recommended portions.

Friendly forums
Members-only forum, providing support, advice and encouragement in a secure, warm, cosy and fun environment – you'll make loads of new low-GL friends here and the authors post regularly too!

Newsletter
Bi-monthly members' newsletter with the latest GL news and research, newly tested foods, new recipes, success stories, healthy eating advice, competitions, goodies and gossip!

Recipe database

Hundreds of low-GL recipes for all tastes with new recipes added each week.

Discounted 'one-to-one' dietetic consultations

Either face to face in Harley Street or by phone with our team of highly respected, qualified, registered dieticians led by Nigel Denby.

Diet plan templates and tools

For when you need a little more help.